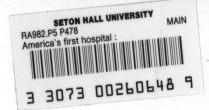
DATE DUE

07/17/96	

GAYLORD PRINTED IN U.S.A.

America's First Hospital: The Pennsylvania Hospital, 1751-1841

By WILLIAM H. WILLIAMS

HAVERFORD HOUSE, *Publishers*

Wayne, Pennsylvania

To my Mother and Father

Acknowledgements

Many people and institutions have made contributions to this book. Of particular significance was the advice and encouragement of four people: John A. Munroe, H. Rodney Sharp Professor of History at the University of Delaware; Whitfield J. Bell, Jr., Librarian of the American Philosophical Society; Richard W. Foster of the Rittenhouse Book Store, Philadelphia; and Joyce Cooper of the Pennsylvania Hospital.

Others who aided this project include George F. Frick, Stephen M. Salsbury and Maynard P. White of the University of Delaware; Robert Brunhouse of the University of South Alabama; John H. Woodward of the University of Sheffield; Norman Capener, Vice President, Royal College of Surgeons, London; Dolores Ziff of the Pennsylvania Hospital; and Ethel O'Connor, former librarian of Delaware Technical and Community College, Georgetown. Fellowships and grants from the American Philosophical Society, the Barra Foundation, and the University of Delaware helped pay some of the writer's expenses. The American Philosophical Society made available microfilms of the early records of the Pennsylvania Hospital.

In addition to the A.P.S., the Pennsylvania Hospital, the Historical Society of Pennsylvania, the British Museum, the Wellcome Institute in London, and the Morris Library of the University of Delaware have been particularly cooperative. Of course a prerequisite to this entire project was the support and encouragement of my wife, Helen.

WILLIAM H. WILLIAMS
Georgetown, Delaware
Dec. 10, 1975

Contents

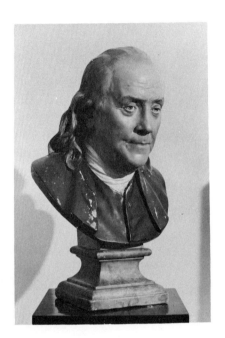 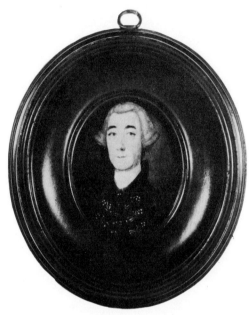

BENJAMIN FRANKLIN   DR. THOMAS BOND
THE FOUNDERS

Our towering modern medical centers seem light years removed from Anglo-America's first hospital, founded in Philadelphia in 1751. And yet, like the equine descendants of some great Arabian sire, the present-day American voluntary hospital can trace its evolution back to its progenitor —the Pennsylvania Hospital. This study focuses on the early years of the Pennsylvania Hospital because it was then, that the institution at Eighth and Pine had its greatest impact on American medicine and philanthropy.

Chapter 1

Genesis

On March 18, 1731, Benjamin Franklin's *Pennsylvania Gazette* featured an appeal to its readers to exercise "a tender regard" for those afflicted with disease. The Philadelphia paper justified this "tender regard" by citing the example of the Good Samaritan and by appealing to enlightened self-interest. But no mention was made of the need for a hospital in Philadelphia or anywhere else in the thirteen colonies.

On August 8, 1751, the *Gazette* printed the same appeal verbatim, with an additional three paragraphs praising even further the example of the Good Samaritan, reporting on the growing hospital movement in Europe and, most important, relating with "a great pleasure," that plans for a hospital had "met with such encouragement in Pennsylvania . . . that there is reason to expect it may be carried into execution the ensuing year."[1] Somehow, in the twenty-year interlude separating the two issues of the *Gazette*, colonial Pennsylvanians, and more particularly, colonial Philadelphians, came to the realization that a hospital was a necessity.

Colonial Philadelphia

Although founded more than fifty years after Boston and almost sixty years after New York, Philadelphia was the fastest growing city in the thirteen colonies. In 1730 her population numbered 11,500, by 1750 she was approaching 15,000, and by 1776 her 40,000 residents made Philadelphia the second largest English-speaking city in the British Empire.[2] Philadelphia's increasing population was supported by a growing economic vitality that made Penn's city the entrepôt, not only for the Delaware Valley, but for a vast hinterland that extended inland, via the Philadelphia Wagon Road, as far as the Shenandoah Valley of Virginia. The docks and wharves along the Delaware teemed with activity as ships bound for the West Indies loaded up with flour, meat and lumber while newly arrived vessels from Great Britain, Ireland, Madeira or Lisbon discharged their cargoes of manufactured goods and wines. Foreign visitors commented with envy on colonial Philadelphia's growing prosperity, but an observing eye would also have noted that certain social problems, miniscule or nonexistent with the first years of setlement, grew apace with the population. The most salient social problem was poverty.

Observers found few traces of either great wealth or real poverty in

1

early Philadelphia. But as Penn's city moved toward the mid-eighteenth century, both wealth and poverty increased in geometric proportions. The ranks of Philadelphia's paupers were dramatically augmented by the large numbers of Scotch-Irish and German immigrants, who poured into the city from 1736 to 1750. In 1749 alone, some twelve thousand Germans disembarked in Pennsylvania. A "large proportion" of the newcomers were "aged, impotent, diseased," or were "convicts and vagrants."[3]

Poor relief in early Pennsylvania was primarily out relief. In 1729, however, the first almshouse in Philadelphia was constructed on Walnut Street by Quakers; but those receiving relief were restricted to impoverished members of the Society of Friends. In 1731 or 1732—the early records have been lost—Philadelphia built a brick almshouse on a square bounded by Spruce, Pine, Third and Fourth Streets. Although, undoubtedly, some medical aid was dispensed to the sick inmates of the Philadelphia Almshouse, this institution's primary function was not that of a hospital. The increase in the number of paupers soon taxed, to the limit, the facilities at the Almshouse, as pauperism continued to vex Philadelphians with no real answer to the problem in sight. Quaker merchant and Assemblyman John Smith made, what was probably a typical observation, in the winter of 1748, when he noted: "It is remarkable what an increase in beggars there is about town this winter—many more than I have before observed. . . ."[4]

The increasing problem of pauperism was compounded by physical and mental disease. Although colonial America's urban centers were probably healthier than their European counterparts, the New World was no disease-free utopia. As Richard Shyrock has pointed out, the thirteen colonies served as a melting pot for diseases, where "Europeans, Africans and Indians engaged in free exchange of their respective infections." Mental illness was also a serious problem to colonial Pennsylvanians. In January of 1751, the Pennsylvania Assembly received a petition which pointed out that "persons distempered in mind, and deprived of their rational faculties hath greatly increased in this province. . . ." The alarm sounded by the petitioners came as no surprise to the members of the Assembly. Legislator John Smith, for example, observed that three Quaker worship services he had attended in the last half of 1750 were interrupted by lunatics.[5]

Faced with increasing numbers of the poor who were suffering from physical maladies and increasing numbers of Pennsylvanians of all classes suffering from mental illness, certain Philadelphians and other Pennsylvanians sought a partial solution to the problem by founding a hospital.

Founding the Hospital

The idea for the Pennsylvania Hospital originated with Philadelphia physician Thomas Bond. A Calvert County, Maryland Quaker by birth, Bond moved to Philadelphia where, in 1742, he was read out of the Phila-

delphia Monthly Meeting. In 1738, in order to further his medical education—the thirteen colonies had no medical school at the time—Bond
embarked for Europe. Although very little is known of his European
activities, we do know that he spent some time in London and at the
famous French hospital, the *Hotel-Dieu* in Paris. Bond probably did not
receive a medical degree while in Europe but he must have profited from
his experiences, having met with some of the most distinguished French
and English physicians and surgeons. In 1739, Bond returned to Philadelphia and two years later was appointed Port Inspector for Contagious
Diseases, a position that must have pressed home the need for an institutional solution to the problems of Pennsylvania's sick-poor.

Benjamin Franklin was a long-standing friend of Thomas Bond's.
Their relationship was further strengthened as the two worked together
to create voluntary organizations, aimed at the improvement of self and
society. Bond joined Franklin's Junto in 1734, and seven years later became a member of Franklin's Library Company of Philadelphia. The two
friends united with others in founding the American Philosophical Society
in 1743 and the Academy of Philadelphia in 1749; the latter an institution
that evolved into the University of Pennsylvania.[6] Obviously, Thomas
Bond shared Franklin's confidence that civic improvement could be
brought about through the efforts of voluntary organizations.

About the end of 1750 or the beginning of 1751, Bond "conceived the
idea of establishing a hospital in Philadelphia for the reception and cure
of poor sick persons . . ." He went about, asking for financial contributions to support his projected institution. But since the idea was a novelty
on this side of the Atlantic and therefore, not understood, Bond met with
little success. He was often asked whether he had consulted Franklin
about his proposed hospital and what did Franklin think of it? When
Bond admitted that he had not consulted with Franklin, his listeners
usually said that they would consider subscribing but would not subscribe at that time. Bond then went to Franklin with his problem, explaining that he had not done so earlier because it was "rather out of your
line . . ." Bond went on to point out that he had found that "there was
no such thing as carrying a public-spirited project through without . . .
[Franklin] being concerned in it." Franklin then asked Bond about the
details of his scheme and upon receiving "a very satisfactory explanation,"
became a subscriber and strong supporter of the Pennsylvania Hospital
Moreover, Franklin's backing was enough to convince many others that
Bond's projected hospital was worthy of support.[7]

By January 20, 1751, a petition in Franklin's handwriting—although
not signed by Franklin—bearing thirty-three names, had been presented
and read to the Pennsylvania Assembly. The petition noted that although
the laws of colonial Pennsylvania had "made many compassionate and
charitable provisions for the relief of the poor, . . ." that something further should be done "in favour of such, whose poverty is made more

miserable by the additional weight of grievous disease from which they might easily be relieved. . . ." The petitioners went on to say that they hoped that the Assembly would share the opinion that a small provincial hospital was necessary.[8]

On January 28, the petition had a second reading and the petitioners were directed to present the Assembly with a bill for a hospital. Within a week the Assembly heard the first reading of a bill "to encourage the establishing of an hospital for the relief of the sick poor of the Province and for the reception and cure of lunaticks. . . ."

The hospital bill met with some objections from rural members of the Assembly because they were skeptical that there was solid, provincial-wide support for the hospital since a hospital in Philadelphia "could only be serviceable to the city." This was a very serious turn because private subscriptions to support the hospital were "beginning to flag." At this critical juncture Franklin saved the day with a clever plan. In order to counter the claim that the general populace did not support the building of a hospital in Philadelphia, Franklin told the Assembly that the pro-posed hospital was in such favor among Pennsylvanians that £2,000 would would be raised by voluntary subscription. The objecting legis-lators considered Franklin's claim "a most extravagant supposition and utterly impossible." Franklin responded by asking permission to submit a second hospital bill that not only incorporated the petitioners but also cleverly stipulated that as soon as £2,000 was raised through voluntary contributions, the Assembly would grant an equal sum to the proposed hospital.[9]

Members of the Assembly who had opposed the first hospital bill were quite confident the Assembly would never have to make the £2,000 matching grant because the hospital's supporters wouldn't succeed in raising the required £2,000 in voluntary contributions. Thus, the reluc-tant rural legislators, thinking "that they might have the credit of being charitable without the expense," agreed to the passage of Franklin's hos-pital bill. As Franklin had hoped, the promise of the Assembly's matching grant provided an additional motive to give, and soon brought in sub-scriptions above the required £2,000. So pleased was Franklin with the way his strategy worked out that he later stated:

> "I do not remember any of my political manoeuvres, the success of which gave me at the time more pleasure: or that in after-thinking of it, I more easily, excused myself for having, made use of cunning."[10]

By early February, 1751, the hospital bill had passed through the As-sembly and Quaker legislators Israel Pemberton, Jr., and John Smith were sent to confer with Lieutenant Governor James Hamilton in order to get the latter's necessary approval. Hamilton had some objections to the bill and insisted on nine amendments before he would sign it. The Assembly was agreeable to all but his seventh amendment, which demanded that the Lieutenant Governor, as well as the Assembly, appoint the "visitors" who would examine the Hospital's "books, accounts, affairs and economy thereof . . ." Realizing that the Assembly was particularly adamant in its unwillingnes to accept amendment seven, Hamilton finally retracted it and on May 11, 1751, signed the hospital bill.[11]

the one on P. 2 bottom *and They gave £2000*
for funding, building & furnishing

Organizing

On July 1, 1751, the Contributors to the Pennsylvania Hospital—all those who contributed £ 10 or more—held their first meeting at the State House. There were some thirty-six people in attendance including such Quaker grandees as Israel Pemberton, Israel Pemberton, Jr., Joseph Fox, John Reynell, Jacob Lewis, Joseph Morris, Anthony Morris, Charles Norris, John Smith and Samuel Rhoads. Among the not-so-wealthy Quakers present was Anthony Benezet, while probably the most notable non-Quaker, besides Franklin and Thomas Bond, was the Provincial Secretary and Councilor, the Reverend Richard Peters.[12]

The Board of Managers

The charter of the Pennsylvania Hospital provided that the Contributors would meet annually in Philadelphia and elect "twelve fit and suitable persons of their own number to be managers of the said . . ." Hospital and one other person to be treasurer. In addition, the Contributors had the right to make all necessary laws and regulations pertaining to the Hospital. At that initial meeting on July 1, the first Board of Managers was elected and given the power to:

> Call a general meeting of the contributors as often as they shall find necessary and that they be desired to prepare such laws or rules as will be immediately wanting.[13]

The very next day the Managers met at Widow Pratt's Tavern—subsequently a favorite meeting place—and, after touring Philadelphia in search of a site for their Hospital, decided to ask Proprietor Thomas Penn for a suitable piece of property. After meeting to elect Joshua Crosby president, and Franklin secretary of the Board, the Managers sent a delegation headed by Israel Pemberton, Jr., to present a request for a suitable plot of land to the Lieutenant Governor. Hamilton responded by stating that he thought that Thomas Penn, if he chose to support the Hospital at all, would give "a sum of money in like manner as others had done." The Lieutenant Governor did, however, write a letter to the Proprietor in which he forwarded the Managers' request and spoke favorably of the Hospital. Not satisfied with entrusting their request for land to Hamilton, the Managers wrote directly to the Proprietor and called on London Quaker merchants Thomas Hyam and Sylvanus Bevan to act as intermediaries with Penn on the Hospital's request.[15] But trans-oceanic communication took months, so the Managers turned to other, more pressing problems while they waited for a reply from Thomas Penn.

The Assembly's matching grant of £ 2,000 was to be specifically applied to "funding, building or furnishing" the Hospital. The more than £2,000 already raised through subscriptions and secured by penal notes, was referred to as the capital stock and, according to the Hospital charter, had to remain inviolate so that it could generate interest and rent to pay the costs of caring for sick-poor patients. In subsequent years the capital stock increased dramatically through contributions from a number of different sources, but the restriction on its use tied the hands of the Managers whenever the Hospital was faced with financial emergencies. If this restrictive stipulation were violated by the withdrawal of funds from the capital stock, the Hospital's charter could be revoked.[16]

Faced with the need to produce income from the principal on hand, the Managers immediately looked for interest-producing opportunities. Initially, short term ventures were favored. On August 20, the very wealthy Israel Pemberton, Jr., offered to borrow £1,000 at "lawful interest." Soon other Managers and other Pennsylvanians followed the example set by the "King of the Quakers." By June of 1752, interest on loans had brought in almost £200.[17]

The First Site

In early September, Managers Joshua Crosby, Thomas Bond and John Smith were chosen to explore the possibility of opening the Hospital in a private home while a new Hospital structure was being planned and built. The committee reported that John Kinsey's house, located on the south side of Market Street below Seventh, was very suitable and could be leased. A Quaker and Speaker of the Assembly, Kinsey had died in 1750. Upon his death it was discovered that this eminent Friend and powerful Pennsylvania politician had bilked the General Loan Office of £3,000. In a frantic attempt to save Kinsey's reputation and to preserve his house from auction, his executors, who included Israel Pemberton, Sr., were eager to see the Hospital rent Kinsey's home. On October 14, after inspecting the house, the Board agreed to the rental at £40 per year and to put £25 into repairs. The rent was to commence as soon as the Hospital was outfitted and the Board guaranteed rental for at least eighteen months, with the option to continue longer at the same rent.[18]

The First Staff

Staffing the temporary Hospital quarters was the next priority. On the same day that the Managers agreed to rent Kinsey's home, Israel Pemberton, Jr., and Thomas Bond were directed to look for a suitable matron to "take care of the house and the sick that shall be placed there." In November, Quaker widow Elizabeth Gardner was hired as matron and in February of 1752, William Sweeting was employed to handle the insane patients, while Alice Courtnet joined the permanent staff as maid and nurse.[19]

Back in February of 1751, when the Hospital bill was first read before the Assembly, some objections had been raised to paying the Hospital's physicians and surgeons because their salaries "would eat up the whole of any fund that could be reasonably expected to be raised." Drs. Thomas and Phineas Bond and Lloyd Zachary met this complaint by offering to attend the Hospital gratis for three years. The three physicians repeated their offer to the Board in October and, on behalf of the Managers, Joshua Crosby happily acecpted and requested that five other Philadelphia physicians "assist in consultation on extraordinary cases."[20]

But What Type Patient?

January of 1752 dawned with the Hospital's matron in control of an empty house; with the capital stock lent out at interest; with three physicians offering their services gratis; and yet no patients had been admitted. But before the admission of patients, it was necessary to adopt specific rules for their regulation, and to state in greater detail the responsibilities and prerogatives of the Managers. To this end a five-man committee of the Board was appointed to draft a general set of regulations. By early January, 1752, the proposed regulations were approved by the Contributors and, as the Hospital charter required, by Chief Justice William Allen, Speaker of the Assembly Isaac Norris and Attorney General Tench Francis.

The new regulations spelled out much more specifically than did the Hospital charter, the powers and limitations of the Board of Managers. Among other prerogatives, the Managers were given "the power to direct the manner and terms of receiving and discharging patients."[21] Spurred on by the necessity of starting the Hospital as soon as possible, the Board turned to the admission and regulation of patients.

The Managers decided to refuse admission to three types of patients: 1. All those judged incurable except lunatics. 2. All those suffering from small pox, "itch or other infectious distemper" until proper apartments were built. 3. Women with young children unless the children were taken care of elsewhere. In addition, those wishing admittance to the Hospital had to provide burial or travel deposits to

indemnify the hospital, either from the expense of burial in case they die, or to defray the expense of carrying them back to their place of abode, that they may not become a charge to the city.

While this last stipulation seems an almost insurmountable barrier to the admission of the sick-poor, the problem was more apparent than real. Local authorities and philanthropists, as well as individual Managers and Hospital staff members, often provided the necessary burial and travel deposits in individual cases. The Managers also decided that if several patients with equally urgent cases applied to the Hospital and there wasn't room for all, preference was to be given to those recommended by the Contributors to the Hospital.[22]

With the exception of the last regulation, admission criteria at the

Pennsylvania Hospital seem to point up the fact that Anglo-America's first hospital was established to aid, indiscriminantly, all of the sick-poor as long as they suffered from a curable, noncontagious malady. But a closer examination of the origins of the Pennsylvania Hospital and, particularly, of antecedent British voluntary hospitals, sheds new light on the type of patient that the Pennsylvania Hospital wished to serve.

The Pennsylvania Hospital was a conscious copy of the British voluntary hospital, as it developed in provincial centers outside of London. These voluntary hospitals were spawned by a reform movement that swept Great Britain during the eighteenth century. The institutions, thus founded, differed from the older Royal Hospitals in that the former were maintained entirely by voluntary subscribers and attended by consulting physicians, gratis, while the latter received support from both municipal government and voluntary subscribers, and used salaried physicians on their staff.[23] Britain's first voluntary hospital was established at Westminster in 1720, but more important to the Pennsylvania Hospital was St. George's established at Hyde Park in 1733. St. George's was the prototype for the first English provincial voluntary hospital founded at Winchester in 1736. The Winchester institution, in turn, became the prototype for most of the subsequent provincial hospitals.[24]

There is no doubt that the founders of the Pennsylvania Hospital had in mind the creation of a "small provincial hospital" of the Winchester type.[25] Franklin's *Pennsylvania Gazette,* in an effort to promote the local undertaking, cited the successful examples of the voluntary hospitals at Hyde Park, Bath, Edinburgh, Liverpool, Exeter and, of course, Winchester. The *Gazette* even carried some information on Anglican clergyman Alured Clarke, the founder of the hospitals at Winchester and Exeter.[26]

Acquiring specific information on the newly founded provincial hospitals, whether at Winchester or elsewhere, was no great problem to colonial Philadelphians. The *Gentleman's Magazine,* published in London but widely read in the colonies—Franklin thought it the best of England's published magazines—carried detailed accounts of individual hospitals. In 1736, it announced the opening of the hospital at Winchester and followed up, in the next year, with a detailed account of that institution's first year. The *Gentleman's Magazine* ended its report on Winchester (often referred to as Hants) by noting that "so truly charitable an undertaking is worthy the immitation of all counties in Britain." Further praise for the Winchester hospital appeared in 1739 and then, in 1741, the *Gentleman's Magazine* published a very detailed account of the new county hospital at Exeter. Subsequent issues carried details of other newly established hospitals including those at Bristol, York, Bath, Reading and Northampton.[27]

Information was also available on British hospitals through numerous hospital reports published by the individual institutions. The first report from Winchester appeared in 1737, and by 1744 Dr. Philip Doddridge, a nonconformist divine, was able to look over published reports of at least five provincial hospitals while in the process of planning the new voluntary hospital at Northampton.[28] Although there is no proof that these published reports were in the hands of the founders of the Pennsylvania Hospital at that institution's inception, there is reason to believe that the supporters and Managers of the Philadelphia institution made a conscious effort to collect published reports put out by the various British hospitals.[29]

Newspapers also carried many reports on the voluntary hospitals in Great Britain. In 1749, for example, an unidentified letter writer noted that the hospital at Edinburgh had been much in the newspapers lately.[30] Certainly many of these newspaper articles made their way to Philadelphia. Philadelphians touring Great Britain supplied yet another avenue of information. A case in point was Dr. Phineas Bond, Brother of the founder of the Pennsylvania Hospital and later one of that Hospital's first physicians, who returned from Europe in 1743 after spending some time in London and Edinburgh. Although there is no extant supporting evidence, it seems safe to presume that the Philadelphia physician toured the important hospitals of those cities and reported to his brother what he saw.[31]

Philadelphians were receptive to the idea of a voluntary hospital because the Quaker city suffered some of the same problems and exhibited some of the same attitudes found in British provincial centers. The growing number of sick paupers was a trans-Atlantic phenomenon as was the Christian impulse to give to those who were less fortunate. Indeed, the example of the Good Samaritan was often called upon to rally support for the voluntary hospitals on both sides of the Atlantic,[32] and more often than not the deeply devout occupied the front ranks of the movement. Quakers John Bellers and Henry Hoare, Anglican divine Alured Clarke and nonconformist clergyman Philip Doddridge, who were front and center in the British voluntary hospital movement, had their Philadelphia counterparts in Quakers John Reynell and Israel Pemberton, Jr., and Anglican clergyman Richard Peters.

The drive for increased medical knowledge also led to support for new hospitals on both sides of the Atlantic during the eighteenth century. As early as 1714, John Bellers called attention to the potential of hospitals in the field of medical education, an argument taken up by Bishop Seeker (the future Archbishop of Canterbury) and echoed in Philadelphia by Franklin's *Gazette* when it pointed out that hospitals

"not only render the physicians and surgeons who attend them still more expert and skillful, . . . but afford such speedy and effectual instruction to the young students of both professions, who come from different and remote parts of the country for improvement, that they return with a more ample stock of knowledge in their art, and become blessings to the neighborhoods in which they fix their residence."[33]

Physicians and surgeons were particularly cognizant of this aspect of the hospital movement and were leaders, in many cases, in the founding of new hospitals. John Harrison in the founding of St. George's, the Royal College of Physicians of Edinburgh in the rise of that city's Royal Infirmary and, of course, Thomas Bond in the founding of the Pennsylvania Hospital are just a few cases in point.

But neither Christian charity nor the growing desire for medical knowledge can wholly explain why the voluntary hospital movement suddenly blossomed on both sides of the Atlantic during the eighteenth century. Rather there was some other aspect of the movement that elicited the same strong support in both Winchester and Philadelphia.

The poor and how they should be treated were much on the minds of eighteenth century Anglo-Saxons. With the increase in beggars and other dependents, poor rates were bound to increase, much to the consternation of the middling sort and their betters. But, noted Alured Clarke in 1737, the antidote is at hand. The hospital, Clarke argued, "will considerably lessen the poor rates in every parish." The same theme was sounded by other hospital supporters, but in greater detail. Poor rates, it was argued, would decline because the hospital was more efficient and therefore less costly than such previously used methods as hiring physicians to treat the sick-poor at home at public expense. By contrast with the older practices, pointed out the Rev. Richard Grey, the care of the sick-poor in a hospital would be only a tenth as expensive. The refrain was picked up in Philadelphia by the *Gazette* which agreed with Grey that the difference in cost was "at least ten to one."[34]

In 1743, the *Gentleman's Magazine* pointed out that if a poor laborer died from medical neglect, his wife and children became a burden to the parish. It was obvious, therefore, that saving the sick-poor was essential on purely fiscal grounds. Eleven years later Franklin seemed to be alluding to this very same point when he noted that a hospital allowed the sick-poor to "became useful to themselves, their families and the public for many years after."[35] Being useful meant, in part, keeping off the poor rolls and therefore keeping down the poor rates. The latter goal was very much on the minds of mid-eighteenth century Philadelphians and contributed to the incorporation of the Overseers of the Poor in 1749 as well as to the founding of the Pennsylvania Hospital two years later.[36]

As the poor increased in number their betters began to express a feeling of uneasiness about the future of the social order. At Winchester, in 1736, Alured Clarke pointed out that the hospital was a means of procuring the affections of the poor and softening their passions. At Northampton, in 1744, the Rev. Richard Grey was even more to the point when he noted that hospital care will

"tend to give the poor in general grateful and honorable sentiment of and inspire them with proper love and reverence towards their superiors, . . . and by consequence promote that harmony and subordination in which the peace and happiness of society consists."[37]

To insure that British sick-poor were aware of their debt to the respective hospitals and, more important, to those who supported those institutions. Discharged patients were required, upon release from the hospital, to offer formal thanks to the managers or governors for treatment rendered. Across the Atlantic the same practice was followed, as the founders of the Pennsylvania Hospital required discharged patients to

> "sign certificates of their particular cases and of the benefit they have received in this hospital to be either published or otherwise disposed of as the managers may think fit." [30]

More central to the rise of voluntary hospitals than the drive to keep down poor rates, or the desire to render the poor more content with their lot, was another aspect of the attitude of the non-poor towards the victims of poverty. In her study of the English poor during the eighteenth century, Dorothy Marshall noted a decreasing sympathy for paupers. Disciplining the lazy and extravagent was advocated with greater energy than previously with workhouses and contractors the expedients proposed and employed. Complaints were often heard of the ill management of private charities "which are too heavily felt to need any particular explanation, . . ." and public laws enacted for the benefit of the poor were merely dismissed as being ineffectual. In Winchester, it was charged, large sums of money given to charity were so misused "that a great many families are known to live in idleness, on the support they receive from the public and private contributions, which are frequently found here. . . ." [39]

Pennsylvania Hospital spokesman Benjamin Franklin was of the same mind. Franklin criticized charitable institutions aimed at aiding the poor because they made the poor "less provident." The giving of mankind

> "a dependence on anything for support . . . besides industry and frugality during youth and health, tends to flatter our natural indolence, to encourage idleness and prodigality, and thereby promote and increase poverty, the very evil it was intended to cure: thus multiplying beggars instead of diminishing them." [40]

Nor did Pennsylvania's Quakers seem much more interested than Franklin in supporting large institutions that would alleviate the sufferings of the poor. Although, in the latter half of the eighteenth century, Pennsylvania's Friends would lead the way in charitable ventures of an institutional nature, in 1751 recipients of organized Quaker benevolence along the Delaware seemed to be largely restricted to those of the Friendly persuasion. [41]

In short, an apparent paradox existed. A trans-oceanic society, ostensibly unsympathetic to institutions aiding the poor, simultaneously spawned a number of voluntary hospitals which, quite obviously, were aimed at aiding the impoverished. A closer look at the situation, however, indicates that rather than a paradox, the founding of the Pennsylvania Hospital as well as the founding of the many British provincial hospitals was a logical outgrowth from this lack of faith in the established methods of dealing with poverty.

The Industrious Poor

English society had distinguished between various types of poor since the sixteenth century. Although the distinctions might vary, generally two subgroups were recognized: those who could work but wouldn't; and those who would work but couldn't. The members of the former group were often referred to as "vagabonds" or "sturdy beggars," while the latter group included the indigent elderly and the dependent young. A third subgroup which would later be labeled the "industrious" or "worthy poor" was also beginning to be recognized by the sixteenth century. Like Gaul, the British poor were divided into three parts.

Relief for the poor was aimed at providing particularly for the elderly and the young via almshouses, orphanages and apprenticeships. As already pointed out, however, sometimes the "vagabonds" and "sturdy beggars" were unwittingly supported by charity.[42] Exasperated because the poor rolls featured lazy but able paupers, it was only logical that eighteenth century Great Britain turn to workhouses to force the reluctant poor to work. In Philadelphia, Franklin applauded the concept of the workhouse as it was being applied in Great Britain and suggested that Pennsylvania needed the same sort of institution. Franklin's main concern was to encourage the "work ethic" (i.e., industry and thrift) among able-bodied colonists, because "as matters now stand with us care and industry seem absolutely necessary to our well being, they should therefore have every encouragement we can invent. . . ."[43]

While the leaders in the British voluntary hospital movement generally castigated the lazy-poor as an unjustified burden to public and private charity, they did single out the "industrious poor" for praise. Encomiums for the latter group reached a crescendo in 1748 when the Rev. John Nixon called them "the strength and bulwark of the nation."[44] The irony of it all was that eighteenth century British charity rarely aided the industrious poor, because that group was self-sufficient and, therefore, "not entitled to a parochial relief." Some of the "industrious poor" even tended to be "ashamed to receive any constant assistance from the parish collections. . . ."[45] Obviously the "industrious poor" were most deserving, but how to help them without further aiding the lazy-poor?

In 1741 the *Gentleman's Magazine*, in an article concerning the "many peculiar advantages of public hospitals," pointed out that unlike other charities, the hospital is not subject to imposters because they would "be discovered by the physicians and surgeons." Moreover, while the profligate and lazy were being weeded out, care would be given to the "multitudes" who had not come under the

> "care of a parish or workhouse; and yet are most of all entitled to the regards of the public, since they are in present want, and are of the diligent and industrious, which is the most useful and valuable part of all society."

Four years later at Northampton, the Rev. Thomas Holme assured his listeners that the voluntary hospital benefited not only society in general, but in particular "those most useful members of it, the industrious poor." Holme went on to say that only deserving objects would be provided for in that hospital and "lazy and clamorous poverty will find no relief." Other voices joined in to inform the public that the new voluntary hospitals were particularly aimed at aiding the industrious and hard working poor.[46]

It was obvious from the beginning that many more sick-poor would apply to the new voluntary hospitals than those institutions, given the limited number of beds available, could admit. Knowing that they would have to be selective with hospital applications, the founders of most British institutions gave a great deal of control over admissions to a governing body chosen by the contributors. (An exception to this generalization was the Royal Infirmary of Edinburgh.)[47] Given the prejudices of the day against "beggars" and "vagabonds," the prospective hospital patient had best produce a good character reference as well as curable, noncontagious illness, compounded by poverty.[48]

A vital first step in the process of establishing voluntary hospitals in Britain had been the recognition that there were "industrious" and, therefore, "worthy" poor. There is some evidence that eighteenth century America was moving in the same direction. In New York, in 1769, it was argued that to assist the industrious poor was not charity but justice, and a study of Philadelphia during the 1790's found a distinction being made in the press between the industrious or worthy poor on the one hand and the "vicious" and lazy poor on the other. This distinction, however, was not universally made in eighteenth century America and the founders of the Pennsylvania Hospital, with the exception of Franklin, did not speak to this subject. Franklin did deal at some length with poverty but, in most of his correspondence and publications, did not distinguish between the industrious and lazy poor. Indeed, through Franklin's eyes "industrious" and "poor" would have seemed mutually exclusive terms since poverty was largely the product of idleness and extravagance.[49]

And yet, on one occasion, Franklin seemed to recognize that some of those suffering poverty did possess praiseworthy traits. The first few words of the act to establish the Pennsylvania Hospital, justified the Hospital on the grounds that it would save and restore "useful and laborious" people to the community. Since these "useful and laborious" people also had to be poor in order to qualify for hospital admission, the words of the act indicate that its author and supporters were sensitive to the fact that some of Pennsylvania's poor were not lacking in industry. As previously noted, the author of the act was Benjamin Franklin.[50]

The act establishing the Pennsylvania Hospital made plain that the purpose behind the founding of that institution was to provide, specifically, for the "laborious" sick-poor. This is understandable in view of the fact that industry and thrift were, in all probability, even more highly esteemed among Philadelphians than among the supporters of voluntary hospitals abroad. Franklin, of course, stands out as the great exponent of the "work ethic," but the other leading supporters of the Pennsylvania Hospital, such as Quaker merchants James and Israel Pemberton and John Reynell, were of the same mind.[51]

In order to assure that the Pennsylvania Hospital's avowed purpose to provide for the "useful and laborious" poor was carried out, a screening process was set up whereby each prospective patient was required to procure a letter signed by an influential person describing his case. As previously pointed out, under certain conditions, patients recommended by Contributors to the Hospital were to be given first preference to the limited beds available.[52] As in Great Britain, charity of this type demanded deference as well as good character on the part of the applicant since his admission depended on recommendations from his betters. Those sick-poor who were turned away from the hospital probably turned to municipal almshouses for succor. A random comparison of patients at the Philadelphia Almshouse (House of Employment and Bettering House) and the Pennsylvania Hospital, during the late eighteenth century supports this assumption. On a typical admission day in 1794, for example, the Philadelphia Almshouse discharged one patient it described as "one of the worst kind," a second who was labeled "a skulking fellow" and a third laconically characterized as "worse." Typical of Almshouse admissions that year was Nathaniel Cope,

> "another of those worthless scoundrels who there is no possibility of keeping in or out and who continually makes a meer slipper of this institution to their own conveniency."

Although a few of the Pennsylvania Hospital's Patients were of the caliber of a Nathaniel Cope, on the whole they seemed a better sort than most of the rabble who ended up in the Philadelphia Almshouse.[53]

As initially pointed out, the founding of the Pennsylvania Hospital can be best seen as an extension of the British voluntary hospital movement to the "New World." During the eighteenth century, the reluctance of the British middle and upper classes to support the older, more established forms of charity was reconciled with self interest and a genuine desire to help the "industrious poor." The voluntary hospital movement met with strong support because it avoided some of the pitfalls experienced by the older forms of charity and, at the same time, served to benefit the "industrious" or "worthy" poor, a group that British philanthropy had hitherto ignored. There were, of course, many other reasons given for the support of the hospital movement—the *Gentleman's Magazine* listed more than ten—[54] but the main impulse grew out of a desire to help, in particular, those poor who showed a decent respect for the "work ethic." It was in the same spirit that Anglo-America's first hospital was created.

Paying Patients

Although the Pennsylvania Hospital drew its founding impulse from the same social forces that produced the voluntary hospital movement in Great Britain, Anglo-America's first hospital did not cater, exclusively, to the industrious sick-poor. The Managers also provided for the admission of paying patients if there was "room in the hospital to spare."[55] Because middle and upper class Pennsylvanians, like their contemporaries in Great Britain, preferred treatment for physical maladies in their homes, paying patients at the Pennsylvania Hospital were generally of three types: indentured servants and slaves whose masters paid the bill; paupers paid for by the overseers of the poor; and the insane from middle and upper class families.

Although paying patients were not usually admitted to the British voluntary hospitals—Edinburg is the one exception that I have encountered—[56] the Pennsylvania Hospital wanted paying patients because they were essential to the Hospital's success. Paying patients maintained middle and upper class interest in the Hospital. With relatives in the cells for the insane or slaves undergoing therapy for serious injuries, some of Philadelphia's merchants were very concerned with conditions in the Hospital. This interest, in turn, led to the demand for better standards than would ordinarily be found in charitable institutions catering exclusively to the poor. Moreover, the availability of an institution that would take troublesome cases of insanity out of well-to-do homes and deposit them in the relative seclusion of the Hospital was a highly appreciated godsend for many emotionally hard pressed families. Philadelphia's "better sort" also appreciated an institution that healed, and returned to productivity, household servants and slaves. Because of the admission of these paying patients, a grateful and demanding middle and upper class could be counted on to contribute heavily to support the Hospital. In addition, paying patients were also admitted because they were profitable in themselves. Generally, paying patients were charged in excess of what they cost the Hospital, and the profit thus generated was used to support additional beds for sick-poor patients.[57]

The First Year

On February 6, 1752, John Kinsey's house was ready to accept its first patients. Furnishings and repairs had been taken care of and the Managers advertised for patients in the *Gazette*. Four days later the Overseers of the Poor of Philadelphia met with the Managers in order to gain admission for "sundry sick poor." After rejecting two applicants, on February 11 the Pennsylvania Hospital admitted its first two patients. By April 28, 1753, the Hospital could boast that sixty-four patients had, so far, been received, of whom thirty-two had been cured and discharged, four had been considerably relieved, eight remained and only five had died. "Several outpatients" had also "received the advice of the physicians and the use of medicines. . . ."[58]

All in all, those connected with the Pennsylvania Hospital could congratulate themselves on a good beginning. Nevertheless, there were some dark clouds on the horizon. The Kinsey house was, at best, a stopgap measure which could hardly hold more than twenty patients at a time and there wasn't enough money to immediately begin construction on a new, more commodious building. Relations with Proprietor Thomas Penn were not the best. Meanwhile, events of ominous portent were about to take place beyond the Alleghenies. Shots fired at the Forks of the Ohio, near present day Pittsburgh, would plunge the frontier into war and destroy, for the present, any possibility that the hard pressed Pennsylvania Assembly could scrape up badly needed additional funds for the Pennsylvania Hospital.

Chapter 2

Managing During the Colonial Years

WHEN GOVERNOR HAMILTON wrote to the Proprietor of the Hospital's request for land, Hamilton also noted that

> the project of this Hospital took its rise principally among Friends, who as they say, are desirous of showing that, when they are not restrained by principle they can be as liberal as others . . .[1]

Quaker Involvement

Throughout the colonial period the Pennsylvania Hospital was largely dominated by Friends. More than two-thirds of those signing the original Hospital petition were Quakers, and the first elected Board of Managers featured seven Quakers, one relapsed Quaker and only four who had other religious affiliations. In addition, the first president of the Board and the first treasurer were Friends. Prior to the American Revolution, 57 percent of the Managers who served the Hospital were Quakers. When only Managers who served five years or better are considered— one suspects that the real leadership on the Board would come from this group—80 percent were Quakers. Continued Quaker dominance is further demonstrated by the fact that up to the American Revolution all presidents, secretaries and treasurers—with the exception of Franklin who served as secretary and then president from 1751-1757—were of the Friendly persuasion.

The above figures on Quaker involvement are even more impressive when considered against the backdrop of a relatively declining Quaker population base. By 1750, only a little more than 25 percent of Philadelphia's population were Friends. Although Quakers were much better represented among the ranks of wealthy Philadelphians—more than half of those who paid a tax in excess of £100 in 1769 were Friends— the power that Quakers exercised over the Pennsylvania Hospital was out of proportion to even their representation among Philadelphia's well-to-do.[2]

While Quakers on both sides of the Atlantic were attracted to the voluntary hospital movement because it offered aid, in particular, to the industrious sick-poor, there were rather unique conditions in Pennsylvania that gave added incentive to Quaker involvement.[3] In 1751 there was some anti-Quaker feeling abroad in Pennsylvania because of the

17

Quaker-dominated Assembly's refusal, on principle, to vote money for the defense of the Pennsylvania frontier. Hopefully, Quaker support for the Hospital would assuage some of this bitterness and improve the Quaker image by showing that "when not restrained by principle they can be as liberal as others."

Perhaps equally important in attracting Quaker support for the Hospital was the obvious evidence that Quakers were becoming, with every year, a smaller and smaller minority in Pennsylvania. The fact had to be faced that Friendly dominance of the Assembly, based on a dwindling population base, could not go on forever. But, as Sydney James has pointed out, Friends could continue to influence public affairs through voluntary organizations.[4] The latter course of action became increasingly attractive to the Friendly community after many Quaker politicians withdrew from the Assembly in 1756, ending the long-held Quaker-dominance over that body.

Thomas Penn and the Hospital

But in 1751, Friends were still in control of the Assembly. Over the previous twenty-five years, growing hostility and distrust had developed between the Penn family and Pennsylvania Quakers, manifesting itself in clashes between the Quaker-dominated Pennsylvania Assembly and the Proprietor over respective political prerogatives. Between 1750 and 1753, Proprietor Thomas Penn attempted to reestablish executive (proprietary) authority in Pennsylvania only to be met by a legislative counterattack spearheaded by Quakers.[5] The chartering of the Pennsylvania Hospital must be seen as part of this legislative counterattack in that it represented a move by the Assembly to assert that it, and not the Proprietor, had the primary responsibility for the approval and regulation of new, voluntary organizations seeking provincial funding.

Upon first hearing of the Hospital bill, Thomas Penn was disturbed and wrote Hamilton, in late July of 1751, that he was sorry "to see every bill sent up to you calculated to weaken the executive part of government." Some five weeks later the Proprietor further stated his dislike for the Hospital act because "it does that which should have been done by letters patent here...." Penn went on to criticize the Assembly for not making his chosen representatives the "visitors" to the Hospital and then drove to the heart of the matter by objecting to the Assembly chartering the Hospital because of the Assembly's "intention to add some power to what they already have which is more than is consistent with the good of the people they represent." Even Lieutenant Governor Hamilton was mildly chatised for signing the Hospital bill before first checking with the Proprietor. In the future, Penn wrote, no Assembly bill shall be allowed "til the thing proposed has been communicated to us."[6]

Not content to give his Quaker adversaries an uncontested victory in this matter, Penn launched a counteroffensive. In late September the Proprietor wrote to Anglican priest Richard Peters—the one Hospital Manager who was a supporter of proprietary government—that he would make a counter proposal concerning the chartering of the Hospital which, if accepted, would lead to a grant of money along with the desired land.

In the spring of 1752 the specific outline of Penn's counter proposal began to take shape. First: London intermediaries Hyam and Bevan reported to the Managers that Lieutenant Governor Hamilton had been directed by the Proprietor to grant the Board's request for land, but not the plot the Managers wanted. Subsequently, the particulars of the Proprietor's instructions to Hamilton were further spelled out. The Proprietor demanded that the Board accept a new charter, granted this time by the Proprietor, in return for a building site. The new charter would give the Proprietor the right to reject or accept any "by-laws, rules and orders" made and approved by the Managers and the Contributors of the Hospital. It would also grant the Proprietor the right to appoint the annual "visitors" (inspectors) of the Hospital, the same right that Hamilton had briefly demanded before relenting to sign the Hospital bill in May of the previous year.[7]

The Proprietor's strategy was quite clear. He would offer a building site to the Hospital, and if that institution rejected his offer, the Proprietor could not be accused of refusing aid to a benevolent institution. Moreover, the plot of land offered to the Hospital lay on the north side of Sassafras, between Sixth and Seventh Streets and was, according to some Philadelphians, part of a square that had been given to the city for public use by William Penn. Acceptance of this public land by the Hospital would reestablish the right of proprietary government to dispose of the remainder of the square in any fashion that it saw fit.[8]

The Managers were displeased with Penn's offer. Not only was there some question concerning Thomas Penn's ownership of the proffered piece of land, but the land itself was judged swampy and unhealthy, and therefore unfit for a hospital site. Particularly galling was the last part of the Proprietor's proffered charter which contained a reversion clause stating that if the Hospital failed and its Contributors ceased meeting, "then the said tract of land thereby granted, shall revert and return to us. . . ." Bothered by the vision of the Proprietor claiming ownership of all Hospital buildings constructed on the donated site, the Managers decided that even if there were no other objections to the Proprietor's offer, the reversion clause was such an objectionable matter that they still "would not entertain the least thoughts of accepting the charter."[9]

When viewed against the larger political issues of the day and the resulting personality clashes, it becomes obvious that the Proprietor's offer would have been rejected no matter how attractive he made the proffered charter. At stake was the obvious question of the Assembly's right to charter and then exercise control over the Hospital. But what made the issue even more difficult to compromise was the personal antagonism that had developed between powerful Hospital Manager Israel Pemberton, Jr., and Thomas Penn.

Although he served only briefly in the Assembly, Pemberton continued to influence the dominant Quaker party's strategy in that anti-proprietary body. Increasingly frustrated over the Quaker party's intransigence, Thomas Penn grew to detest and fear Israel Pemberton. When Pemberton was not returned to the Assembly after the election of 1751, Penn jubilently exclaimed his pleasure and went on to label Pemberton "the most turbulent creature that has appeared in the Province." It is no wonder that Penn was reluctant to grant autonomy from proprietary control to an institution that was under the influence of such a "turbulent creature."[10]

Although Theodore Thayer, Pemberton's biographer, maintains that the King of the Quakers "entertained no personal animosity toward the Penns of his generation . . ." one suspects that a man of Pemberton's volatile nature would strike back at his political enemies with any means at hand. As an influential Manager of the Hospital, as well as a director of the Quaker party's struggle against proprietary government, Pemberton was bound to view with suspicion any move made by the Proprietor. Moreover, most of the other Quakers on the Hospital's Board were members of Pemberton's social circle and, therefore, subject to his influence. In short, the Hospital was not only in the hands of Quakers, it was under the influence of the least compromising faction of that sect. If Isaac Norris or other less rigid Quakers were as influential in Hospital affairs as Israel Pemberton, perhaps an accommodation could have been reached with the Proprietor. That, however, was not the case and an amiable relationship between the Proprietor and the Hospital was just about impossible during that institution's first few years.[11]

Although Penn's proposed charter had been rejected by the Managers, the original Hospital charter had yet to receive the necessary royal approval. If Thomas Penn used his influence with certain prominent men in court, George II might be persuaded to veto the charter. Intermediaries Hyam and Bevan, after presenting the Proprietor with the Hospital's rejection of his proffered charter, found Penn quite incensed at the Hospital's actions. But at this point Thomas Penn's professed concern for the welfare of Pennsylvania seems to have overridden his mistrust of Pennsylvania's Quakers. On October 26, 1752, Penn wrote Hamilton that the Hospital Managers' objections to his offer, and particularly to the reversion clause, "showed that they were not in earnest . . ." but nevertheless, he had recommended to the Privy Council that the Hospital charter be approved by the crown because "I would not object to any law you [Hamilton] had passed." A day later Penn wrote Richard Peters: "I have presented the Hospital act and think to let it pass with the others." On May 10, 1753, the Hospital act, along with eleven other acts passed by the Pennsylvania Assembly, was ratified by George II.[12]

Although he offered no resistance to crown approval of the Hospital act, Thomas Penn continued to brood over his rude treatment at the hands of the Assembly and the Hospital's Board of Managers. Nevertheless, in 1754, the Proprietor, in a moment of charitable enthusiasm, declared that he would give the Hospital an annual sum. Within a few years renewed hostilities between the Proprietor and Israel Pemberton, centering primarily on a disagreement over Indian policies, again strained relations between the two and no grant was made by Penn nor would he sell the plot originally desired by the Hospital.[13]

In 1762, with the Hospital's first decade proclaimed a grand success, Thomas Penn was finally able to overcome his earlier reservations and favored that institution with a generous grant. After hearing good accounts of the Hospital from William Logan and others, Thomas Penn, together with his brother Richard Penn, agreed to contribute £40 in Pennsylvania currency "on the first day of May and on the same day every year until further orders." During that same spring the Penns offered to grant to the Pennsylvania Hospital the remainder of the square bounded by Pine, Spruce, Eighth and Ninth Streets not already owned and occupied by the Hospital. The £40 contribution was paid annually up to the American Revolution and the patent for the donated plot was finally delivered in 1767.[14] The fact that by 1762 Benjamin Franklin, not Israel Pemberton, represented the greatest threat to proprietary government may have influenced Penn's decision. Perhaps it was fortunate for the Hospital that Benjamin Franklin had relinquished his official ties with that institution in 1757.[15]

A New Hospital at Eighth and Pine

Once the Hospital Act was approved by the Crown, the Managers were able to plan for the future with a great deal of confidence. In 1754, because Judge Kinsey's house was only a stopgap measure of limited utility, the Board turned again to seriously considering the purchase of a building site. A committee of four phsicians and six Managers viewed several possible locations and within two days agreed to buy the lot belonging to the Free Society of Traders in Pennsylvania, which covered part of the square bounded by Eighth, Ninth, Spruce and Pine Streets. On December 7, 1754, the deed was turned over to the Hospital after that institution borrowed the £500 purchase price from its capital stock.[16]

Prior to the purchase of the building site, the Board discussed plans for a new hospital structure, and builders Samuel Rhoads and Joseph Fox were directed to draw up plans for the proposed structure, after consulting with those Contributors who were skilled in building. Both Rhoads and Fox had begun their adult lives as carpenters or builders, although since that time both men's financial interests had broadened considerably. After consulting with the Contributors and physicians, and laying before the Managers the plans of the Royal Edinburgh Infirmary in Scotland, Rhoads and Fox presented a rough plan for the new hospital in late January of 1755.[17] Thanks to an engraving printed by Robert Kennedy in 1755, the exterior of the proposed structure is available for our scrutiny.[18]

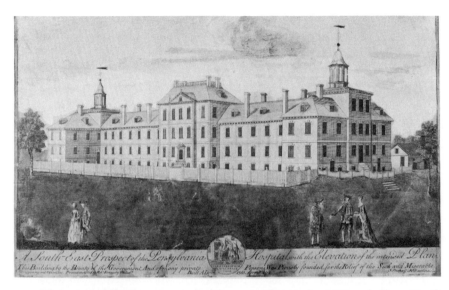

The general design was probably more the work of Rhoads than Fox[19] and featured two T shaped wings, mounted by identical cupolas, joined together by a central building topped by a balustrade. The two wings were to be two and one half stories while the balustraded center portion was to be three and one half stories. Here indeed was unornamental functionalism[20] combined with a typical eighteenth century respect for symmetry. Each of the three sections was functionally independent in itself and yet, when finally completed, the three sections would form a harmonious whole. During the last decade of the eighteenth century the Board of Managers saw fit to make some changes in the details of Rhoads' grand design. Nevertheless, by the completion of the total structure in 1804, the Pennsylvania Hospital stood, in part, a monument to the architectural and building skills of Samuel Rhoads.

It is difficult to trace the genesis of Rhoads' Hospital design. The exterior of the projected structure does not seem to have been copied from any one contemporary building. Yet it is quite clear that the overall hospital design was subject to the considerable influence of the British voluntary hospitals in general, and the Royal Infirmary of Edinburgh in particular. It is not too difficult to link such concepts found in the Pennsylvania Hospital plan as the operating room and gallery in the attic, the wards on either side of a central building and the cells for the insane on the ground floor, to the example of the Edinburgh infirmary design.[21] But then, it is only natural for the Pennsylvania Hospital to look to the Edinburgh infirmary for example. In 1754 the Scottish hospital served a populace only a little larger than Philadelphia, and provided for the mentally as well as the physically ill. Moreover, the consulting architect of the Edinburgh infirmary, William Adam—father of noted architects James and Robert Adam—drew up plans for a large structure with only one section to be constructed immediately. The remainder of the Edinburgh Infirmary was to be completed as soon as the requisite funds were available. By 1748, the infirmary's building program was complete, giving Samuel Rhoads a concrete example to draw from.[22] Although Rhoads designed a structure "on a larger scale than anything hither-to attempted in the colonies, . . ."[23] only the eastern third of the building was completed in his lifetime. It was to this structure that Rhoads turned his immediate attention.

On February 22, 1755, a month after submitting his rough plan for the entire structure, Rhoads laid before the Managers a detailed plan for the eastern wing of the Hospital. The Managers decided to call the Contributors into meeting on March 10, at the Court House, so that Rhoads' plan and the estimated expense could be laid before them.[24] The Contributors, upon being presented with the plan, which would cost an estimated £3,000, unanimously approved and authorized the Managers to proceed with construction as quickly as possible. After conferring a considerable time, the Managers unanimously chose Samuel Rhoads to provide the materials and superintend the construction. It was also decided that any subscribers who were "workmen" could be employed in

> "doing as much work at least as the amount of their subscriptions, provided they be ready when called upon."

Evidently, just as in the British voluntary hospital movement, some of the supporters of the Pennsylvania Hospital expected business advantages in return for benevolent giving.[25]

On March 15, eight of the Managers viewed the recently purchased lot and unanimously agreed that the south front of the eastern wing be set back one hundred-fifty feet from Pine Street and the east front of the wing to be sixty feet from Eighth Street. The location of a pump and well was fixed at the northeast corner of the wing. On May 28, the Managers invited the treasurer and the physicians to accompany them to see the foundation laid. Schools in the city were dismissed and a large crowd assembled at the site of the new structure. The cornerstone, engraved with the appropriate words of Benjamin Franklin, was laid with Masonic rites. On October 27, the Board adjourned its meeting for one hour to attend the "raising of the roof of the wards of the new building." Thirteen months later (November 29, 1756), it was announced that the new Hospital was just about ready for occupancy.[26]

Plans for the impending move from Judge Kinsey's house were quickly formulated and carried out. Joseph Kinsey, an heir to Judge Kinsey, was notified of the Hospital's plan to move—the lease on the house expired on January 1, 1757—and a man was hired to start fires in the several fireplaces of the new structure in order to dry it out. The matron was ordered to employ a woman to wash the several apartments in the new building, while the monthly sitting committee was directed to consult with the matron regarding the additional furniture needed in the new structure. On December 17, 1756, the matron moved the patients and furniture into their new home at Eighth and Pine.[27]

To approach the newly constructed east wing of the Pennsylvania Hospital, a visitor would travel westward from the heart of the Quaker City, leaving behind the urban sprawl that marked the fastest growing metropolis in America. The Hospital's setting was certainly bucolic, as shown in an engraving as late as 1768.[28]

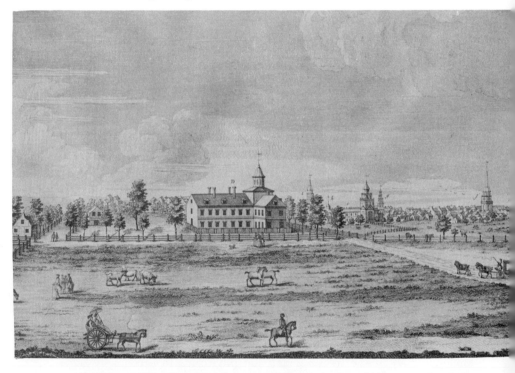

But this isn't surprising, in view of the fact that during much of the eighteenth century, Philadelphia's urban growth pushed north and south along the Delaware River rather than westward. In 1756 the hospital lay four or five city blocks from the edge of Philadelphia's urban sprawl, and it would be the end of the century before the homes and buildings of the Quaker City began to envelop the Hospital's area of Eighth and Pine.[29]

Once he had made his way over unpaved roads to Eighth Street, our visitor would observe that the ground plan of the lone structure facing him looked like an inverted "T." Climbing the entrance steps to the first floor, he would find himself in a long hall, running from left to right, that led to a consultation room, an apothecary shop, and apartments for the steward, matron and other staff. Directly across the hall, making up the leg of the T, lay the men's ward which was eighty by twenty-seven feet with windows on both sides providing optimum ventilation. A large walk divided this ward with rows of beds on each side. Above lay the second floor, basically of the same design, with a female ward and smaller rooms along the hall for private patients and "such who cannot be admitted in safety into the grand wards." In the basement, below the men's ward, the leg of the T was divided into cells for the insane with a gallery down the middle, while the remainder of the basement was occupied by baths, the kitchen and pantry. A little distance from the main building stood a wash house, stable and garden.[30]

For a number of years after the first patients moved into the new building, some of the interior work remained unfinished. On March 21, 1759, the Board called for the completion, as soon as possible, of

"the unfinished cells, the paving in the cellars, and the north and east fronts of the house."

By May of 1759, various members of the Boards were personally undertaking certain finishing touches on the cells and front steps, but a year later work was still continuing on the same projects.[31]

Nor was the lag in the completion of the building the only complaint. A few of the craftsmen employed were heavily criticized for cheating the Hospital. John Gilchrist and John McCauley did not

make the steps to the front door according to agreement made with them last year when ten pounds was advanced to them towards the work.

The complaint against Gilchrist and McCauley was lodged in 1758, but these same steps continued to be a source of irritation to the Board for some years. Finally, in 1763, a stone cutter supplied stones for the steps but at a cost of £72.4.3, a price which appeared "very extraordinary," and a committee was assigned to get the cost reduced.[32] There is no indication that Samuel Rhoads was the focus of any of this dissatisfaction. The trouble was merely the same found in contracting with local craftsmen anywhere; a few are bound to prove unreliable and even dishonest.

The Board of Managers

The new building was not the only concern of the Managers. Although the physicians were often consulted, and their advice sometimes listened to, essentially the broad outlines of policy, the control of financial affairs and the approval of further physical renovations were exclusively the prerogatives of the Board, subject, of course, to the approval of the

Contributors. Because of the Board of Managers' significance, it is necessary to take a closer look at that body as it existed down to the American Revolution.

The Contributors—all those who contributed £10 or more to the Hospital—annually elected twelve of their number to serve as Managers for the ensuing year. The Board usually met at least once a month, and sometimes more often, if there were pressing business. If one of the Managers resigned or died in office, the remainder of the Board chose a successor to fill the vacant seat until the next annual election, which was always held in May. During the first Board meeting in May, usually a week after the yearly Contributors' meeting, the Managers held annual elections for president and secretary. The only other non-salaried officer of importance was the treasurer, who was also elected annually, but by the Contributors.

In objecting to the Pennsylvania Hospital's Charter, Thomas Penn had been wary of that charter's apparent democratic tendencies which gave "every subscriber of ten pounds . . . a right to give his vote."[33] In the case of the Pennsylvania Hospital, however, the majority of eligible voters did not bother to cast their ballots at the annual elections for the Board of Managers and the treasurer. In 1754, when there were approximately one hundred twenty-nine Contributors, only sixteen cast their ballots at the annual election in May. With each year, the number of Contributors showed a sizeable increase, and yet voting participation did not show a corresponding climb. Although, after 1754, the actual number of Contributors in any given year is impossible to accurately ascertain, it is obvious that only a small fraction bothered to cast their ballots. The last pre-Revolutionary War figure on Contributor voting indicates that only twenty-four ballots were cast. In a few annual meetings, more Contributor interest was shown—in 1766, forty-one votes were cast, to mark the high point of participation—but overall the Contributors did not seem to take their voting responsibility very seriously.[34]

One explanation for Contributor apathy was that Board election results were a foregone conclusion.[35] Elections were decided ahead of time by that same small coterie of men who made most of the decisions for the Pennsylvania Hospital down to the American Revolution. Year after year the same family heads were reelected to the Board of Managers or to the position of treasurer without any challenge to this oligarchical system. In short, Thomas Penn's fears of anarchic democracy controlling the Pennsylvania Hospital seem ill founded in view of events up to 1776.

While that small coterie who exercised such strong control over the Hospital did not exclude non-Quakers from election to the Board, those Managers who were non-Quakers tended to be anti-proprietary Anglicans.[36]

An exception was the election, in 1751, of Richard Peters, a sometime Anglican priest who worked for Thomas Penn as Provincial Secretary as well as serving as a member of the Provincial Council. Strongly attached to the Proprietor, Peters was upset by the Board's treatment of Thomas Penn in 1751 and refused to sign the Board's initial request to the Proprietor for a hospital building site. Thomas Penn was well pleased with his employee's actions but the Board must have been irritated by this early show of disharmony. Five years later James Pemberton would indicate Quaker impatience with Peters by referring to him contemptuously as "the old priest Peters," but for the year 1751 and 1752 the Quaker talent for understatement and the desire to keep the sympathy of some Anglicans probably explains the lack of open reference to Peter's intransigence. Through the winter of 1751-1752, Richard Peters was noticeably absent from meetings of the Board and in May of 1752, his name did not appear on the list of reelected Managers.[37] With Peters no longer on the Board, a new sense of unity prevailed because now the Managers could present a completely united front to the Proprietor.

Not surprising, in view of the antagonism between Quakers and Presbyterians, was the absence of "Convenanters" from the Board of Managers. William Allen, the leading Presbyterian layman in Philadelphia and the Chief Justice of Pennsylvania, contributed more money than any of the Quaker grandees to the Hospital, but was never elected to a Hospital position. One of the few "Convenanters" to be elected to the Hospital Board during the colonial period was Daniel Roberdeau, who, unlike William Allen, was anti-proprietary in his politics. In 1756, he was strongly supported by Quaker Israel Pemberton in a successful campaign for election to the Pennsylvania Assembly.[38]

To summarize briefly, the Managers had a certain religious-political unity that set them apart from a normal cross sampling of Philadelphians. If the Managers were not all of the Friendly persuasion, they did share the common denominator of anti-proprietary political views. Of course, when some of the Quakers abandoned their anti-proprietary position in the early 1760's, this common denominator ceased to exist. Nevertheless, it did last long enough to provide a unifying adhesiveness to the Board of Managers during those very crucial early years. By 1765, James Pemberton, brother of Israel, noted that the Hospital Board was rent with "divisions" and "opposite sentiments," but the tradition of unity established in earlier years was such that

"the attention and care for promoting laudable purposes of this useful institution remains uninterrupted." [39]

It is not possible to categorize the occupations of the Managers into neat, meaningful units due to the diverse nature of most of their incomes. Some, such as Samuel Rhoads and Joseph Fox, started as builders but soon branched out into real estate and mercantile activities. Others such as Israel Pemberton, turned from mercantile adventure to real estate. Most were probably interested in both real estate and the import-export trade. All were wealthy men who accepted the social responsibility of their status. While some, such as Franklin, were "nouveau riche," the majority, like the Pembertons, represented at least two generations of wealth.[40]

Most Hospital Managers could be found in other benevolent or civic improvement organizations. The Philadelphia Almshouse, the Union Fire Company and, the Friendly Association for dealing with the Indians, were among the groups served by members of the Hospital Board.[41] One exception to this tendency of the Managers to serve on other civic organizations can be found in the case of the College of Philadelphia, because that institution was a rallying point for the Anglican proprietary forces just as the Hospital served as a rallying point for the Quaker anti-proprietary group.[42]

Because of the Friendly desire for anonymity, it is difficult to decide who were the most significant members of the Board during the colonial period. However, a number, through their long years of service and their membership on crucial committees, stand out. Significantly, the likes of Joshua Crosby, Israel Pemberton, Benjamin Franklin, Samuel Rhoads, John Reynell, and Hugh Roberts were serving from the very inception of the Hospital. Of the Managers elected later, only James Pemberton, Isaac Greenleaf and Thomas Wharton would exercise a like influence over the fortunes of that institution.

Joshua Crosby served as president of the Board until his death in 1755. Because he was the presiding chairman, Crosby should be given some credit for the smooth functioning of the Hospital in its first four years. His membership on so many key committees, and a death legacy of £100, testify to the commitment of this Quaker merchant to the Hospital. In order to fill Crosby's position, the Managers turned to Benjamin Franklin.[43]

Some of Franklin's earlier contributions have already been mentioned. Throughout the colonial period, Franklin's *Pennsylvania Gazette* carried timely notices of Hospital news and events. Meetings of the Contributors were advertised and the election results reported. Even lists of subscribers were published, along with their contributions, causing consternation in at least one quarter. In 1771, an embarrassed donor complained that

> "when I compare that small sum which I have given, to several of those mentioned as aforesaid, I confess I should almost be ashamed to see my name, on account of the poor figure it would make with some of those in the last list of contributors. . . ."

The writer went on to say that the whole affair prejudiced his disposition to give to the Hospital.[44] Despite the embarrassed contributor's lament, it was very helpful to have the free publicity of newspaper articles, whenever necessary. Moreover, the relationship was beneficial to both parties involved. The Hospital received free publicity and Franklin and

Hall received printing business, in return, from the Hospital. In 1766, for example, the two partners were paid £81 by the Hospital for services rendered.[45]

Franklin served only two years as president of the Board and then left for England. It is difficult to evaluate Franklin's leadership during this period but one fact is inescapable; Franklin rarely attended Board meetings from September of 1756 to April of 1757 when he embarked for England.[46] While in England, Franklin continued to serve the Hospital in a number of ways, not the least of which was the simple strategem of telling others of the benevolent institution fronting on Eighth Street in Philadelphia. In his *Autobiography*, Franklin again stated his high regard for the Hospital, but when He returned to Philadelphia in later years, he never again sat on the Board of Managers, nor was his will as generous to the Hospital as Joshua Crosby's.[47]

Once the Hospital was launched, Israel Pemberton, the "King of the Quakers" became the key figure. Within the Friendly fold, Pemberton was a towering figure who had little use for democratic methods. The oligarchical control which dominated Quaker meetings demonstrated that wealth was synonymous with leadership,[48] and Pemberton and his fellow Quakers brought this principal into the Board of Managers' meetings. In session after session of the Board and in the Contributors' annual meeting, unanimity seems to have prevailed because Israel Pemberton and a few others dictated proceedings as they had done at Quaker meetings

Only once during his long career as Manager, which stretched from 1751 to his death in 1779, do the Hospital's archives disclose that Israel Pemberton did not get his way. In January of 1760, the majority of the Board was intent upon hiring George Weed as steward-apothecary, but Israel Pemberton and two other Managers dissented. By May of that year the other two Managers had changed their minds leaving Pemberton alone in opposing Weed's employment. With the overwhelming approval of the rest of the Board, Weed was hired, and Israel Pemberton's position of leadership had been challenged.

The election of the Managers that May reflected the "King of the Quakers" fall from favor as he received only twenty-three votes, seven less than the number garnered by most of the other Managers. Subsequently, Pemberton regained his position of leadership and in the following year's election no Board member received more votes. As if to vindicate this new vote of confidence, Pemberton turned increasingly to Hospital work at the cost of other activities. By 1765 the "King of the Quakers" had relinquished the clerkship of the Yearly Meeting and declined other offices in order to concentrate on Hospital affairs as well as on some other humanitarian interests.[49] Not the least of Israel Pemberton's contributions to the Hospital was the interest he aroused among English Quakers in the brick structure at Eighth and Pine. The leading

American Quaker was aided in this task by his brother James, who became an important Manager in his own right.

James Pemberton was younger than Israel and exercised less influence in the Quaker community. In 1758, James Pemberton was elected Manager of the Hospital and continued to be reelected until his retirement in 1780. From 1759 to 1772 the younger Pemberton served as secretary of the Board, keeping up a steady correspondence with English Quakers concerning the Hospital. It might be expected that James Pemberton would defer to his older brother on important issues but this was not always the case. On the question of the appointment of George Weed, for example, James Pemberton voted against his older brother's position.[50]

Samuel Rhoads continued to serve as the chief advisor on construction and repair problems. In 1780 Rhoads was elected president of the Board, only to go into retirement the following year. In 1774, in a brief vignette, a contemporary portrayed the Quaker builder as

> "a respectable merchant of Philadelphia, belonging to the Society of Friends—without the talent of speaking in public, he possessed much acuteness of mind, his judgement was sound and his practical information extensive."[51]

Also well thought of by his peers was Quaker merchant John Reynell, who was elected the first treasurer of the Hospital in 1751. The following year Reynell was elected to the Board and subsequently served as president from 1757 until his retirement in 1780.[52] Others who stood out as Managers in the colonial period included Thomas Wharton (1762–69, 1772–79),[53] Isaac Greenleaf (1756–1771), and Hugh Roberts (1751–56). In addition to serving as Managers, Roberts and Wharton were elected treasurers, the former from 1756 to 1768 and the latter from 1769 to 1772. All of the above mentioned Managers were Quakers with the exception of Franklin and it was easy enough to link Franklin with the Friendly persuasion. The French, in later years, referred to him as "Le ban Quaker," and even Ernst Troeltsch mistakenly cited Franklin as a Friend. It is no wonder that Chastellux, on visiting Philadelphia in 1780, implied that the Pennsylvania Hospital was an exclusively Quaker enterprise.[54]

In 1758 Hugh Roberts wrote Franklin that

> a few good and charitable institutions have failed of a support where harmony remained among the Managers and party views were discouraged.[55]

At the time Roberts was treasurer of the Hospital and, no doubt, had that institution in mind when he made his observation. In 1758, factionalism was no threat to the Hospital, as anti-proprietary sentiment was still in the air and, although perhaps less strident than in earlier years, it still served to unite the Board.

But as the American Revolution approached, members of the Board were often at odds on provincial issues—James Pemberton had indicated a divergence of political opinions as far back as 1763. Perhaps the most significant intra-Board political clash took place in 1769 between Israel Pemberton and John Reynell over the proper reaction to the Townshend Acts. Reynell led a boycott movement against British imports while Pemberton led a movement in the Society of Friends to condemn Reynell's activities. Reynell's group subsequently moderated its position, and soon after, the Townshend duties were repealed. Despite this difference of opinion, there is no indication of strained relations between the two leading Quakers during Board meetings.[56]

Finances

The finances of the Pennsylvania Hospital from 1751 to 1775, although punctuated at times with fiscal emergencies, generally featured the continual growth of the Hospital's capital stock (see Appendix) and the raising of construction funds to pay for the new building. By 1775 the revenue generated by the capital stock was such that some seventy patients at a time could be housed and treated gratis in that institution.

In colonial Virginia, the managing of one's private circumstances was crucial in deciding fitness for public office because

> a man who could not manage well his own affairs ought not be entrusted with the management of public affairs.[57]

So too did eighteenth century Philadelphians measure a man for a position of responsibility, and the election of the Hospital's Board of Managers reflected this same, seemingly all pervasive, attitude. If an Israel Pemberton could balance well the critical variables of the import-export trade he certainly would see the Hospital through to sound financial footing. Indeed, the public equation of private success with qualification for public trust—although technically a private corporation, the Pennsylvania Hospital essentially functioned as a public institution and therefore the office of Manager was a public trust—was very clearly justified in the case of the Managers because of their constant attention to the Hospital's financial affairs. Patients were admitted, prescribed to and operated on, nursed, and, hopefully, discharged cured. But all of this cost money, and the Board had the responsibility of producing the same through public appeals for funds, and then, the careful investment of surplus funds in income producing ventures.

Initially, the Managers depended on Franklin's *Pennsylvania Gazette* to advertise the Hospital's good works and need for financial support; but in 1753, in need of more cash to finance their new building, the Managers decided that some added publicity was necessary. On May 5, 1753, Franklin was directed

> "to prepare a full account of the affairs of the Hospital . . . to be laid before the Assembly."

Franklin went on to write *Some Account of the Pennsylvania Hospital*, which covered the history of that institution from its inception to May of 1754.[58]

Typographically, the first edition of *Some Account* was Franklin at his best. In content it represented as much didactic eclecticism as objective history; but no wonder since the primary purpose was to gain public support. On the last page of his forty page account Franklin shrewly provided a contribution form to make immediate contributions to the Hospital easier.[59] Fifteen hundred copies of *Some Account* were printed in quarto, and by late July, 1754, some issues had already been distributed. With an eye on English subscriptions, a dozen copies were sent to London Friends Thomas Hyam and Sylvanus Bevan, with the request that the two Londoners distribute them

> "in such manner as may be of most service, and that if you find any of your friends disposed to contribute towards this good work, you will promote them doing it."[60]

The impact of *Some Account* was soon apparent. By August 4, 1754, the Board reported that several new subscriptions had been obtained since the last meeting and, in a particularly puzzling move, the Board "agreed to be very careful about asking others." Perhaps there was a certain uneasiness among Quakers that non-Quakers might some day form a majority of Contributors or, at least, a troublesome minority. By April of 1755, whether screened or not, the Hospital added 186 new subscribers who donated over £2,000 to the capital stock. In the year prior to the publication of *Some Account,* only one new Hospital subscriber was recorded, pointing up the unusual effectiveness of Franklin's publication.[61]

Franklin's contributions to fund raising did not end with publicity. In 1752, he proposed that boxes be set up to receive Hospital donations. The Board instantly approved the idea and "Hugh Roberts and Samuel Rhoads were appointed to get them made." These charity boxes, placed in homes, the Hospital, and public places, led to impressive results. From 1753 to 1775 they produced over £900 for the Hospital.[67]

In 1759, due to an increase in operating costs and the expenses incurred in completing the new building, the Hospital found itself in financial trouble. Although, according to the Hospital charter, the capital stock was to be left inviolate, the Board got around this restriction through a bookkeeping procedure. Needed funds to cover the deficit in operating expenses were taken from the capital stock with a simple notation that the withdrawn money was owed to that fund. In 1758, for example, the capital stock was listed as £5,052, but because £164 had been transferred that year to meet operating expenses, only £4,888 actually remained in the capital stock. By borrowing from the capital stock, the Board was able to meet short term emergencies. But, in the long run, this practice jeopardized the Hospital's existence. If the capital stock could not be built up to produce a sizeable yearly income—in the hospital fiscal year ending in April, 1758, the capital stock generated only £212, while the household expenses for the same period, amounted to £472—the Hospital could never attain a desirable financial position, and might succumb to a sudden financial reverse.[63]

In March, 1759, the hard pressed Board decided to ask the Assembly for a grant to increase the capital stock. Back in 1751, when the Pennsylvania Hospital had received legislative aid, some of the Hospital petitioners, such as Israel Pemberton and John Smith, were members of the Assembly. But now, because many Quakers had voluntarily withdrawn from the legislature in 1756, there were not as many strong supporters of the Hospital in the Assembly.[64]

But the Assembly was not without some appreciation of the Hospital. A year prior to this new request for funds, it resolved to help support the Hospital by donating fines assessed the Assembly's membership for tardiness.[65] Needless to say these fines—a shilling for each case of tardiness—never amounted to very much. What the Hospital needed from the Assembly was a grant similar to that made in 1751; that is, in the neighborhood of two or three thousand pounds.

On March 28, 1759, the appeal from the Managers reached the Assembly, stating that

> "the Managers have been reduced to the necessity of applying most of the contributions obtained from private persons for these three last years past, towards completing the works [the new Hospital building], which hath of course prevented an increase of the capital stock, the annual interest whereof is the only fund yet established for the support of the institution. . . ."

Financially pressed by war expenditures, the Assembly did not act on the Hospital request for two years. Finally, on September 12, 1761, a committee appointed by the Assembly recommended government funds be voted to aid the Hospital. During the following year the Assembly granted £3,000 to the Pennsylvania Hospital in order to replenish that institution's capital stock.[66]

A few years later, even the commissioners, appointed by the Assembly to pave the streets of Philadelphia, got into the act. Having a surplus of funds on hand and no immediate use for them, the commissioners loaned the Managers £4,000 for one year without charging interest. By investing the £4,000, the Managers were able to add over £360 to the Hospital treasury.[67]

The Assembly's beneficence was matched by renewed support from private contributers, which helped push the capital stock above the £10,000 mark by 1763. This new outpouring of public and private support was stimulated by a tried and true technique: the publication of a Hospital history. Since Franklin was no longer in Philadelphia, a committee of Samuel Rhoads, Isaac Jones, Evan Morgan and James Pemberton produced a second history of the Hospital covering the years 1754 to 1761. By April of 1761 the Managers were in the process of printing their continuation of Franklin's earlier history, and on January 25, 1762, the Managers were informed that over six hundred of the accounts were printed.[68]

Donations made to the capital stock by private investors did not always take the form of currency. As, in the case of the previously mentioned Penn grant, some land was given outright, or even loaned, so that rentals might be collected by the Hospital. Indeed, the first real estate actually owned by the Hospital was a plot of land lying between Philadelphia and Germantown donated by Matthias Koplin in September of 1751. Koplin accompanied his gift with a letter complaining of the abuse of hospital contributions in his native Germany and stating by way of contrast, his confidence in the Pennsylvania Hospital. The Managers reassured Koplin that his gift would be put to good use and

> "as a caution to future managers against such misapplication, they [the Board] have ordered thy letter to be copied in their book of minutes . . . that it may be preserved to posterity, as a testimony of the original intention of the founders of this institution."[69]

Of particular importance to the Hospital, during the colonial years, were the sums of money donated by the signers of Pennsylvania's emissions of bills of credit (a form of paper currency). Currency signers were necessary because numbering machines and facsimile reproduction of signatures did not yet exist. In 1754 the Managers asked the Assembly to allow certain friends of the Hospital to sign new emissions of bills of credit since those same friends promised that the fee paid them by the colonial government would be donated to the Hospital. Nothing came of the proposal in 1754, but in 1757 signers of bills of credit turned £684 over to the Hospital. During the remainder of the colonial period similar donations followed and, by the beginning of the American Revolution, contributions from this source had amounted to about £3,000. Signers who contributed to the Hospital in this fashion were often neither Managers nor Contributors. Thus it seems that by donating the fees produced by the rather arduous task of signing bills—forty-five shillings per thousand signatures was the going rate in 1765—some Philadelphians who had not previously taken an active interest in the Hospital's welfare, now did so.[70]

Gifts from England fulfilled some of the expectations of the Managers. Generous monetary donations from the likes of the very wealthy Quaker merchant David Barclay and the distinguished Quaker physician John Fothergill were gladly received.[71] Sometimes the Board used ingenious means to move reluctant English donors. From the beginning, the Hospital had been purchasing its drugs from the English drug firm headed by Sylvanus and Timothy Bevan. On May 20, 1765, the Managers wrote to John Fothergill that the Bevan brothers had failed "to favour us with a donation from themselves. . . ." In a letter of the same date to the Bevans, the Managers chastised the London Quaker druggists because the last parcel of drugs was much larger than necessary and was "charged at a higher price than we could have bought them here." The Managers went on to chide the Bevans for being in affluent circumstances and yet not contributing to the Hospital. They also took to task all of the merchants of Bristol and London for not allowing a discount on drug sales for indeed "we are informed 10% has been made on such occasions by some druggists." Finally the Managers closed by stating that the list of Contributors to the Hospital was not complete without "your name." Timothy Bevan responded with an offer of five guineas a year—Sylvanus Bevan had passed away in June of 1765—but this gesture did not satisfy the Board. A reluctant Timothy Bevan finally authorized the Board to draw on him for £50 sterling, "a sum thought here a generous donation to any of our great hospitals."[72]

Victory over the Quaker druggists of Plough Court led to the use of like tactics on another of London's Quaker druggists. By 1769, the Managers were again discontented with the prices of Bevan's drugs and decided to meet the Hospital's needs through local purchase. Within a year the Hospital's physicians protested that it was certainly cheaper to purchase drugs from England and an order was again sent off to Timothy Bevan and Sons. Four years later, however, a drug order was sent to a new source in England, one Thomas Corbyn of London, along with a letter requesting a contribution for the Hospital. Corbyn responded that because he had so many charities to contribute to, he would not contribute to the Pennsylvania Hospital, but that his partners had jointly decided to subscribe £100 sterling. Corbyn's associates, hoping no doubt that their donation would contribute to both good will and good trade with the Pennsylvania Hospital, must have been sadly disappointed to receive on May 6, 1775, a note from the Hospital's Managers stating that "the present state of public affairs will not permit . . ." the importation of more drugs.[73]

All private donations from across the Atlantic were eagerly received by the Managers, but the Board was particularly pleased by the Pennsylvania Land Company windfall. The company, located in London, had been formed in 1699 and held property in Pennsylvania, New Jersey and Maryland. In 1760, in order to expedite the sale of land, the company's holdings were vested in nine trustees, chiefly Friends and including Dr. John Fothergill. Many shares of the company had gone unclaimed and, under the urging of Fothergill and Thomas Hyam, Parliament established that after June 24, 1770, all unclaimed shares of the company would be turned over to the Pennsylvania Hospital. Since the nine trustees were selling off the company's holdings, the Hospital would be entitled to a percentage of the aggregate selling price, commensurate with the unclaimed shares.[74]

While the Board searched for an agent to receive the windfall, Fothergill predicted that the Hospital's shares in the Pennsylvania Land

Company would amount to £6,000 or £7,000 sterling. In 1771, after a long delay, the Managers were told by Fothergill that the unclaimed shares of the Pennsylvania Land Company were deposited in the Bank of England waiting "on the execution of a suitable power of attorney." After meeting with the Contributors and receiving the approval of the Pennsylvania Assembly, the Managers empowered Fothergill, Benjamin Franklin and David Barclay to receive any money due the Hospital from the Pennsylvania Land Company's unclaimed shares.

The newly empowered attorneys, however, did not correspond with the Board, and letters were sent to the three pointing out the Hospital's disappointment "at not hearing from them." After more than a year had passed since their appointments, Fothergill, Franklin and Barclay responded that the money was still tied up because of slow progress in obtaining a decree from Court of Chancery. Finally, in August, 1772, the three Hospital agents wrote that the remaining shares of the land company had been transferred to them in the form of bank annuities, but because these securities fluctuated in price, it was hard to report how much they would be worth. Nevertheless, it seems that the Hospital had gained, through the beneficence of Parliament and the hard work of certain individuals, approximately £8,637 sterling.[75]

The Hospital's capital stock had reached £10,000 in 1763, but during the nine subsequent years had increased only slightly. Thanks mostly to the addition of the Pennsylvania Land Company grant in 1773, the capital stock almost doubled to more than £22,000 (see Appendix). But not all of the capital stock represented actual currency. Income producing gifts, such as land and buildings, were given a monetary value and added to the capital stock.

For the sake of analysis, the Hospital's capital stock can be divided into three separate categories. The first category represented currency donated outright by the Assembly or subscribers. The percentage of the total capital stock thus represented, generally increased as the American Revolution approached. Back in 1758, it represented about 60 percent of the total, while in 1775 that figure had grown to 79 percent. The Managers chose to loan this money out on interest, demanding, in good businesslike fashion, substantial security, usually in the form of land, from the borrower. Precedence was layed down as early as 1751, when the Board agreed to loan £300 to Isaac Greenleaf, on the latter giving "clear security in land of at least double the value. . . ." In general, the first category yielded a return of almost 5 percent.[76]

The second category represented the subscriptions pledged with notes, but not yet paid off in cash. Subscribers whose contributions fell into this category, paid an annual interest on the total of the pledge. In contrast to the previous category, these unfulfilled notes tended to represent a decreasing percentage of the capital stock as the years passed. In 1758, this category amounted to 36 percent of the capital stock but by 1775 it barely amounted to 8 percent. It is difficult to assess the income return from this classification, but it probably did not exceed 4 percent.[77]

The third category was primarily real estate, exclusive of the Hospital's buildings and grounds at Eighth and Pine. Valued at 12 percent of the total capital stock in 1775, the third category generated income at the annual rate of between 3 and 4 percent.[78]

But no matter how much income the capital stock generated, the Hospital's annual expenses always kept one step ahead (see Appendix). The household expenses alone—this did not include expenditures on new buildings—increased almost fourfold between 1758 and 1775. And yet, if we look only at the capital stock vis-a-vis the household expenses, the pattern of development was encouraging. In 1759, after two full years in the new building, the Hospital's annual household expenses amounted to 16 percent of the capital stock. By 1775, that figure was down to slightly less than 8 percent. If, by 1775, the Hospital was not 100 percent healthy, at least its financial base was growing stronger each year.[79]

A Little Bit of Pragmatism

If eighteenth century Americans differed from contemporary Europeans in their pragmatic approach to problem solving, the members of the Board of Managers of the Pennsylvania Hospital were among the most pragmatic of Americans. Even George Whitefield, a friend of Franklin's, but certainly not well liked by Friends, was allowed to preach a charity sermon on the Hospital's behalf, in 1764.[80]

But it was in the winter of 1759-1760 that the Managers best demonstrated their practical bent. On December 27, 1759, an advertisement appeared in the *Pennsylvania Gazette* proclaiming that "the celebrated Tragedy of Hamlet Prince of Denmark" would be presented the next day, for the benefit of the Pennsylvania Hospital. Given Quaker opposition to public theatrical performances, and the fact that nine of the twelve Managers were Quakers, one is left with the conclusion that the Board, in its subsequent activities, compromised its religious scruples for the sake of the Hospital. Obviously aware of the performance—one of the non-Quaker members, Evan Morgan, was selling tickets—the Board waited until January 7, 1760, to note what had transpired. By that time the proceeds from the play had been "paid into the hands of the treasurer." Then, assuming an indignation suitable to their position of leadership in the Friendly community, the Quaker grandees expressed their dissatisfaction and demanded that an advertisement be published in the *Pennsylvania Gazette,* declaring that the powers of the Managers are such that

> "they are not authorized to direct the treasurer to refuse the money lately raised by exhibiting a stage play near this city . . ."

even though the said play "was done without the consent of the said

Managers. . . ."[81] Shades of 1745, when the Quaker-dominated Assembly refused to vote military supplies for the expedition of Louisbourg, but voted instead for £4,000 to be laid out for the purchase of bread, meat, wheat, flour, and other grains for the King's service. Franklin said that the governor understood "other grains" as the Quakers intended and therefore purchased the necessary "black powder." The Friendly casuistry of 1759 was hardly unique.[82]

In retrospect, during the colonial period the Hospital's Board had weathered some challenging crises, financial and otherwise. Through firmness bordering on intransigence, through compromise verging on capitulation, by solicitations that were, at times, intimidating, and above all, through hard work and a steady eye on the practical implications of their actions, the Board managed to meet each challenge successfully. But perhaps none of this would have meant much without good luck. The Hospital was lucky in its overseas friends such as David Barclay, John Hyam and John Fothergill.

The fact that the reputation of Pennsylvania Quakers escaped the French and Indian War pretty much intact was another stroke of good fortune, as it permitted the realization of large grants and windfalls from the Pennsylvania Assembly and the English Parliament. Of course, there was the chance that the next decade or even the next year would bring a change of luck, a different throw of the dice. And yet, as Candide would have pointed out, "Cela est bien dit, mais il faut cultiver notre jardin."[83] The physicians and the rest of the staff of the Pennsylvania Hospital had been doing that very thing since 1752.

Chapter 3

Healing During the Colonial Years

The Physicians

ALTHOUGH LLOYD ZACHARY and the Bond brothers had offered to attend the hospital gratis for three years, it was obvious that additional physicians would be needed and that rules for regulating the Hospital's physicians were necessary. In April of 1752, the Contributors adopted a series of regulations that empowered the Managers to choose, each May, six physicians to serve the Hospital for the ensuing year. The six physicians were to serve without salary and were to agree with the Managers on a schedule of attendance. Although Thomas Bond had been elected to the first Board of Managers, the Contributors stipulated that Hospital physicians could not, simultaneously, serve on the Hospital staff and on the Board.

The regulations further stipulated that before a physician could be considered for election to the Hospital's staff, he had to contribute at lease £10 to the Hospital, spend a period of time as an apprentice in the Philadelphia area, spend seven years or more in the study of physic or surgery, and pass an examination presided over by the Hospital's physicians and witnessed by the Managers. Even candidates with impressive foreign credentials had to reside in Philadelphia for three years and pass the required examination before they could be considered for election.[1] What sort of practitioners possessed these qualifications and were attracted to Anglo-American's first hospital during the colonial period? To better answer this question, a brief examination of the colonial physician is in order.

American colonial physicians were not, as a group, possessors of impressive academic credentials. Of an estimated 3,500 practicing physicians in the American colonies in 1775, no more than 400 had attended medical school on either side of the Atlantic.[2] Faced with little educational opportunity in the formal sense—the medical school of the College of Philadelphia, which was the first institution of its type in the thirteen colonies, did not open its doors until 1765—the colonial physician learned his trade through observation and practice. He usually apprenticed himself to an established member of the medical profession and, after a period of years of practical training, went off to set up his own practice. His patients would call him doctor even though no university degree had been earned or a licensing test passed.

In retrospect, it has been argued that the colonial physician's lack of university education, with its emphasis on theory and systems, may well have been a blessing because most theories of medicine, held during the eighteenth century, were incorrect.[3] Only with the theoretical nihilism of the nineteenth century could medicine throw off the fetters of "wrong theory" and begin all over again to ascertain the truth about disease. The greater the academic training of the eighteenth century physician, so that argument goes, the more dogmatic in support of "wrong theory" he became. Thus the graduates of Edinburgh and Rheims and Leyden justified the heroic regimen of bleeding, purging, blistering and sweating on theoretical rather than empirical grounds. One has only to look to the career of Benjamin Rush, a graduate of Edinburgh, for a case in point. Rush urged that patients be relieved of three-fourths of their blood in order to overcome tension. Perhaps a less educated physician would have been less bound to "wrong theory," less committed to such drastic remedies and, therefore, less of a threat to his patient's life.

Argue as we may over the merits of an eighteenth century university medical degree, to most eighteenth century minds it was an asset. In its first medical staff and the ones to follow right up to the American Revolution, the Pennsylvania Hospital felt itself very fortunate. Of the eleven physicians who served the Hospital from 1752 to 1775, at least nine had some medical training abroad, with six receiving M.D. degrees from foreign universities. On the initial staff of six physicians elected in 1752, degrees from Rheims and Leyden were represented. During the remainder of the colonial period, however, all additions to the staff who held M.D. degrees, were Edinburgh graduates.[4] The academic credentials of the Hospital's physicians, if not impeccable, were certainly impressive by the standards of the day.

Although not many colonial physicians had time to publish their medical observations, the staff of the Pennsylvania Hospital was unusually prolific in this area. During the colonial period, Thomas Bond had two papers published by a London medical journal, while Thomas Cadwalader published *An Essay on the Iliac Passion* in 1740 and five years later, an essay on lead poisoning from drinking punch. John Redman published at least two papers by 1759, and Cadwalader Evans' account of using electrical shock treatments to relieve a young woman suffering from convulsions was published in London in 1752.[5] In 1765, John Morgan, a year after presenting the great Italian pathologist, Giovanni Battista Morgagni, with a copy of his thesis on pus formation, published his very significant *Discourse upon the Institution of Medical Schools in America,* which advocated the separation of the functions of surgeon, physician and apothecary and laid before the public his plan for establishing a medical school in the College of Philadelphia.[6] By 1766 the medical school curriculum was established and by 1769 it was staffed by five physicians, who were, or would be, at some future time, physicians of the Pennsylvania Hospital.[7] Obviously the Managers of the Hospital had chosen well, for the practitioners who served the Hospital represented the leadership of their profession in the Quaker City.

The first elected staff of six physicians was composed of the Bond brothers, Lloyd Zachary, Thomas Cadwalader, John Redman and Samuel Preston Moore. They served as a unit until Lloyd Zachary suffered a paralytic stroke in 1753 and William Shippen, Sr., was chosen to fill the vacant position. In 1759, Samuel Preston Moore retired, to be replaced by Cadwalader Evans, while in 1773 John Morgan and Charles Moore were chosen to fill positions left vacant by the deaths of Phineas Bond and Calwalader Evans. The following year Charles Moore retired and his position was filled by Adam Kuhn.[8] Overall, the stability of the medical staff was exceptional with a turnover of only five physicians in twenty-five years.

The eleven Hospital physicians who served during the colonial period were a less homogenous group than was the Board of Managers. While four were Quakers and three others were former Quakers, the Presbyterian, Anglican and Lutheran faiths were also represented.[9]

Political affiliations were likewise varied. Among the anti-proprietary faction was Cadwalader Evans, but strongly supporting proprietary interests was William Shippen, Sr. Although Thomas Bond was personal physician to John Penn and William Allen, he worked hard to keep political antagonism from jeopardizing the progress of the Hospital and the betterment of science and medicine in Philadelphia. Whereas the Managers, with a few exceptions, looked upon the College of Philadelphia as a hostile camp, the physicians of the Hospital were much more favorably disposed toward that "rallying point for Anglicans." Indeed, in 1765 John Morgan pointed out that five of the six attending physicians of the Pennsylvania Hospital were also trustees of the College.[10]

As is so often the case, political differences generated less divisiveness than vendettas generated by personal ambition and professional jealousy. John Morgan, prior to being elected to the Hospital staff, embroiled himself in a dispute with William Shippen, Jr., over which of the two should receive credit for first proposing the medical school in Philadelphia. The Morgan-Shippen dispute began in 1765 and simmered for a number of years. William Shippen, Sr., on the Hospital staff at the time, was, no doubt, drawn into the dispute. Another disagreement concerning Hospital physicians occurred in 1774, when Doctors Morgan, Rush and William Shippen, Jr., attempted to curtail Thomas Bond's clinical lectures which were held at the Pennsylvania Hospital, and were a degree requirement of the medical school. Actually, the reason for the attack on Bond was that the three critics wanted to give the clinical lectures themselves. Adam Kuhn vigorously rallied to Bond's defense and Bond's clinical lectures continued as a requirement for a medical degree from the College of Philadelphia.[11]

Despite disagreements leading to tension between members of the medical staff, personal animosities are not even hinted at in the Hospital's records. In this regard one is reminded of the case of John Hunter, Britain's most famous eighteenth century surgeon, who died, it is said, from a heart attack brought on by a roaring good argument with his colleagues at St. George's Hospital, London, where Hunter was a member of the staff. The couch upon which Hunter died is still preserved in that institution, but St. George's records make no mention of the argument, noting only that J. Hunter, one of the surgeons, had died. Certainly, there must have been a great deal more ill feeling at Eighth and Pine than the records indicate, but the practice of having compatible physicians work together on the two-man attending teams must have reduced tension considerably.[12]

Ostensibly at least, the Hospital's physicians seemed very sympathetic to the plight of the sick-poor. After all, the physicians did work without salary and even provided in a few cases, the necessary burial deposits so that some sick-poor might be admitted.[13] Closer examination, however, paints quite a different picture. Colonial physicians did not treat the sick-poor particularly well because colonial physicians, like other eighteenth century men, were great respecters of a person's social position. Furthermore, physicians regarded their calling as a trade and they did business with those who could pay best. Indeed, the eighteenth century physician's almost callous contempt for the sick-poor comes through with astonishing clarity in a letter from Phineas Bond to Samuel Rhoads. The Pennsylvania Hospital physician reported that he had visited a number of English hospitals,

"where the great variety of sick and lame affords not only matter of instruction but amusement."[14]

As far as legacies were concerned, of the eleven Hospital physicians, only Lloyd Zachary left money to Philadelphia's only institution expressly concerned with the sick-poor. Even the providing of free service was not so much a matter of charity as it was an opportunity. In Great Britain as well as in Philadelphia, physicians served gratis on voluntary hospital staffs because appointment to a hospital position offered both honor and experience which could not be duplicated elsewhere. By contrast to the free service they gave the Pennsylvania Hospital, Thomas Bond and Cadwalader Evans simultaneously served the less prestigious Philadelphia Almshouse; but for a salary of £50 per year.[15]

John Welsh Croskey, partisan historian of the Almshouse, even goes so far as to maintain that Thomas Bond founded the Pennsylvania Hospital in order to find a place "where he could take his more affluent patients where they could pay for services rendered." Crosky was obviously unfamiliar with the records of the Pennsylvania Hospital and unaware of the founding impulses behind the voluntary hospital movement. But his questioning the altruism of the Hospital's physicians creates a counterweight to the eulogistic cant of Pennsylvania Hospital historians Thomas G. Morton, Frank Woodbury and Francis Packard.[16]

Perhaps the fairest way to assess these eleven physicians is to view them in the context of their time and profession. Like other eighteenth century physicians, their main energies were devoted to acquiring experience, preferment and reputation. If there was enough time and energy left over to dispense a little charity as well, all the better. Saints they were not; but then their business was of this world and not the next.

Although the division of the Hospital's medical staff into physicians or surgeons did not officially take place until the early nineteenth century, some specialization took place at an early date. Phineas Bond, for example, did not care much for surgery while his brother became quite adept at it. In November of 1752, Thomas Bond performed the first amputation at the Hospital when he removed Susannah Bromholt's leg. On November 29, 1756, with amputations of legs and breasts by now a not uncommon occurrence in the Hospital, Bond performed what was probably the first lithotomy, not only in the Pennsylvania Hospital, but in the thirteen colonies.[17] John Morgan was also skilled in surgery, having worked as regimental surgeon of the Pennsylvania Provincial troops from 1756 to 1760. Morgan's subsequent views on the separation of the functions of surgery and physic, however, indicate that Morgan disdained surgery while serving as Hospital physician.[18] No doubt the other physicians performed some minor surgery and bled their patients when therapy demanded, but major surgery was pretty serious business— Thomas Bond's second lithotomy in the Hospital led to a patient's death[19] —and, therefore, seems to have been left to the experienced hand of the Hospital's founder.

Insane patients formed a significant part of the Hospital's admissions, and it might be expected that one or two of the physicians would specialize in this area. Although the records are inconclusive, Thomas Bond did seem to have a considerable interest in the mentally ill. While Bond was serving his turn on the admissions committee, a higher than normal percentage of newly admitted patients were suffering from mental diseases.[20]

A typical year for a physician on the Hospital staff meant riding out to Eighth and Pine Streets two days a week—usually the second and fifth days—for four months of the year. Working in tandem with another physician, his time at the Hospital was split between admitting new patients—in conjunction with the two-man committee of Managers—and seeing to the needs of those patients already in residence. Sometimes business or other commitments interferred with this schedule and only one physician would show up. Often the physician would be accompanied by his apprentices as he walked the wards. During the two-thirds of the year that he was not on duty, the Hospital physician still might be called in as a consultant in "extraordinary cases."[21]

During the colonial period, the Managers and the Hospital's physicians seem to have gotten along well enough. After all, if the Board was dissatisfied with any one of its six physicians it could refuse to reelect the offending physician the next year. The fact that the Board never exercised this prerogative from 1752 to 1775 is indicative of the relations between the two groups. This is not to say, however, that the Board-physicians relationship was always tranquil. In 1758, for example, an irritated Board directed the Hospital's medical staff, in the case of patient Henry Adams, to "either pursue some more effectual method of his recovery or that he be discharged." In May of 1770, the Board

> "agreed, that a conference be had with the physicians of last year, on some regulations which appear necessary for the better conducting the business of their department. . . ."

The Board then made a number of demands on the physicians pertaining to the purchasing of drugs; the intrusion, deportment and fees of students; the dissecting of bodies by young surgeons, and control of access to the anatomical paintings and casts donated by Dr. John Fothergill.[22] Although the physicians acquiesced in most of the Managers' demands, they did maintain that the annual student fee of six pistoles, demanded by the Managers, was too high and that the more reasonable fee of £5 be charged. Although it took over three years, the Board finally agreed to a £5 annual student fee.[23]

Despite the instances cited above, the Managers thought that the Hospital's physicians performed in a highly satisfactory manner. In 1762, Manager James Pemberton wrote to John Fothergill that if the present Hospital physicians should resign, replacements could not be found of similar experience and integrity. Earlier that year some of the doctors had proposed to be released

> "from the service in order to give others an opportunity and leave no room for uneasiness to any of the Contributors who might imagine they were re tained through motives of partiality and a desire in them to engross the reputation to themselves."[24]

The Board would not hear of the latter proposal and the reelection of the entire staff of physicians in 1763 expressed the Board's confidence in that body.

Medical Education

One of the most attractive features of the Hospital was its potential as an educational institution. At the Pennsylvania Hospital, as in most British hospitals, apprentices of Hospital physicians were not charged by the Hospital for the right to follow their preceptors through the wards for a first hand look at the havoc wrought by disease, and the counter therapy prescribed. Evidently, apprentices to non-Hospital physicians were also allowed to walk the wards but, beginning with 1763, had to pay a fee for the privilege. Although records of students allowed into the Hospital are only fragmentary, we do know that in the winter of 1765-66, thirteen students including Benjamin Rush, student of John Redman, and William Bartram, son of the noted botanist John Bartram and eventually an outstanding naturalist in his own right, were walking the wards.

Not all students apprenticed to non-Hospital physicians bothered to pay the required fee. In 1770 the Board noted that those students apprenticed to other than Hospital doctors must pay six pistoles for the privilege of attendance, "which for a year or two past hath not been duly observed." The fee price was finally lowered in 1773, and, in at least one case, where the apprentice was too poor to pay, the fee was waived.[25]

Up until 1762 no formal instruction in medicine was offered at the Hospital. The physicians, followed in their rounds by their eager young students, discussed individual cases and were, no doubt, helpful according to the standards of the day; but no lectures were given. All of this was changed by a gift from Dr. John Fothergill in 1762. In April of that year, Fothergill informed James Pemberton that he would send with William Shippen, Jr.,—Shippen was finishing his medical education in Great Britain at the time—a present of "instrinsic value, though not probably of immediate benefit." Fothergill, after stressing the importance of the knowledge of anatomy, added that

"some pretty accurate anatomical drawings about half as big as life have fallen into my hands. . . ."

Fothergill directed that these drawings, along with the several anatomical casts, be used as a basis of anatomical lectures by Dr. Shippen. On November 8, William Shippen, Jr., presented himself before the Board, informing that body that Fothergill's gift to the Hospital had arrived, and requested the use of the drawings in order to "exhibit a course of lectures on anatomy this winter." The Managers granted Shippen this right, provided that the lectures be given in the Hospital, and that each pupil who attended be charged one pistole, the money to be used for the benefit of the Hospital. The idea of charging a fee of any one using the drawings and casts had been Fothergill's suggestion. Shippen did not begin his first lecture until May 21, 1763, and continued them thereafter once every fortnight to "students in physic" as well as to others interested in a "general knowledge of the human body."[26]

As Dr. Fothergill pointed out, "for want of real subjects [cadavers]" the drawings and casts would "have their use."[1] In Anglo-Saxon countries, opposition to the dissection of human bodies survived down to the middle of the nineteenth century. Indeed, the fact that society objected to the use of bodies in this manner, led to such nefarious activities as grave robbing and body snatching.[27] The Quaker City shared this aversion to the "desecration" of dead bodies. It wasn't until 1742 that the first published postmortem examination was undertaken by

Thomas Cadwalader, who would later join the staff of the Pennsylvania Hospital. The Managers of Anglo-America's first hospital, very concerned with the image projected by their institution, were particularly sensitive to the negative impact that dissections at the Hospital might have on public opinion. Thus, in 1770, the Board complained to its medical staff that

> "the indecent conduct of some young surgeons in taking up and dissecting dead bodies, occasions a general uneasiness and displeasure in the minds of all humane people."

The Managers asked the help of the physicians "in remedying this evil." The physicians responded that they would do all in their power to prevent further dissections by the students.[28]

Objections to unruly students carrying on dissections did not, however, preclude the use of cadavers by individual Hospital physicians for instructional purposes. In 1765 William Shippen, Jr., moved his anatomical and obstetric lectures to the new medical school of the College of Philadelphia. For a brief period of time the Hospital's facilities were not being used for formal instruction, although for some time Thomas Bond and some others of the staff had been giving informal instruction, sometimes obtaining a body for the purpose of examination. But clinical instruction of this sort depended almost entirely on the initiative of the Hospital's physicians. Doctors Morgan and Shippen—in 1765 these two were the only instructors offering courses at the new medical school—regarded formal clinical instruction as an integral part of a complete program of medical education. Therefore, the two physicians asked Bond to continue, in a more systematic fashion, his clinical teachings. Bond decided that Board approval of a more expanded program of clinical instruction was necessary and sent that body a letter describing his proposal. Evidently the Board gave an indication of approval, and Thomas Bond invited the Managers and the Hospital's physicians to his home on November 26, 1766, to hear the first, or introductory, lecture that he would deliver that winter.[29]

Thomas Bond's introductory lecture, with its emphasis on post-mortem examinations, is an extraordinary statement. Only five years earlier, the great Morgagni of Padua published his significant *De Sedibus et Causis Morborum*, which laid the basis of modern pathology. In 1764 John Morgan, touring through Western Europe, met Morgagni and received, as a gift, the two volume *De Sedibus*. Perhaps Bond had borrowed *De Sedibus* from Morgan on the latter's return to Philadelphia in 1765. Influenced or not by Morgagni, the full medical implications of Bond's introductory lecture go far beyond the scope of this study. Whitfield Bell, Jr., notes that Bond's lecture ranks

> "second only to Morgan's *Discourse* in importance for medical education in eighteenth century America."

Of direct impact on the Hospital was Bond's rather laconic statement that hospitals "are justly reputed the grand theatres of medical knowledge." In the thirteen colonies there now was a hospital that offered over one hundred live patients for study! But equally important was the examination of the dead, for how else could errors in judgement be rectified "for the benefit of survivors . . . ?" The founder of the Pennsylvania Hospital went on to point out the value of two autopsies performed the previous fall and the Board got the message. Right there in Bond's home, the Managers approved the upcoming clinical lectures, demanded that each student who wished to sit in on the lectures pay one guinea per year, and made provisions for supplying cadavers. The matron of the hospital was directed ot take the bodies

> "of patients who die . . . into the upper hall, to be laid out in a suitable apartment there. . . ."

Whenever Bond or another Hospital physician wished to use a cadaver he had only to ask the consent of the attending Managers.[30]

Attendance at Thomas Bond's clinical lectures was a requirement for a degree from the medical school, and in the ensuing five years, ten to fifteen students were enrolled at a time. Not all of the students thought well of Bond's clinical lectures and indeed, as previously mentioned, student discontent fed by the jealousy of Bond's colleagues led to a crisis in 1774.[31] Nevertheless, Bond's clinical lectures rode out the storm and, until the American Revolution, the Hospital continued to be used to teach one of the medical school's required courses.

The Medical Library

Crucial to the education of both the young students and the older physicians was the development of a medical library. The building constructed on Pine Street had no room for a library, and students were forced to depend upon the private collections of individual physicians for reading material. In 1762 the Hospital received its first medical book when William Logan returned from London, with *An Experimental History of the Materia Medica* by William Lewis, a present to the Hospital from Dr. Fothergill.

In 1763, when the Hospital decided to charge students of non-Hospital physicians for the privilege of walking the wards, the Hospital's physicians seized this moment to write to the Managers that,

> "as the custom of most of the Hospitals in Great Britain has given such gratuities [student fees] to the physicians and surgeons attending them, we think it properly belongs to us to appropriate the money arising from thence, and propose to apply it to the founding of a medical library in the said institution [Pennsylvania Hospital] which we judge will tend greatly to the advantage of the pupils and the honor of the institution."

The Board agreed with the proposal, provided that the Managers approved all books purchased, as well as the manner in which they were lent out. Other student fees, such as those paid for Dr. Shippen's and Dr. Bond's lectures, also went into the library fund.

Despite the vigorous action taken by the Hospital's physicians, no new books were added to the library collection until 1767. In January of that year, two bequests of books caused the Managers to build book shelves in their meeting room, giving the medical library its first official home. Forty-three volumes and some pamphlets were received from the estate of recently deceased Hospital physician, Dr. Lloyd Zachary. A week later Deborah Morris gave the medical library some fifty-five volumes belonging to her late brother, Dr. Benjamin Morris, a graduate of Leyden. Caught up in enthusiasm for the growing library, the Managers authorized Thomas Bond to order more books from England. By the end of November the newly ordered books were on the library shelves. In 1774 the steadily growing library fund allowed another book order to be sent to London and by December of that year a trunk of books arrived, sent by London bookseller William Strahan.

As soon as the library became an established fact, volumes were donated by interested parties. But some of the donated volumes were non-medical in nature and were stashed away in a trunk. The growing library was not without its problems. Evidently, outsiders were in the habit of entering the library, borrowing books and then not returning the same. In 1774, the Managers ordered that books be lent out only to Managers, physicians, and students of the Hospital or of the medical school. Promissory notes or deposits were demanded equal to the value of the borrowed book, and certain valuable volumes could be used only in the Hospital.[32]

The Anatomical Museum

A gift of a human skeleton, in 1757, began the Hospital's fine collection of anatomical materials. In 1762, upon reception of Dr. Fothergill's drawings and casts, the Managers set aside a room to serve as an anatomical museum. In 1772, the museum collection was further enlarged by the addition of another human skeleton and preparations of muscles and arteries purchased from the estate of physician William Logan. The museum room was kept locked with the key in the hands of one of the Managers, and those who wished to examine the exhibits in the locked room were charged a fee.[33]

The Apothecary

Apothecaries, like most colonial physicians, learned their trade by serving apprenticeships. Although most colonial physicians combined the functions of apothecary, surgeon and physician in their practice, the Pennsylvania Hospital, following the example of British voluntary hospitals, recognized at an early date, the desirability of hiring an apothecary. In 1752, Jonathan Roberts became the hospital's first apothecary at a salary of £15 per annum, plus room and board. Roberts was expected to

> "prepare and compound the medicines and administer them agreeable to the prescriptions of the physicians and surgeons . . ."

Roberts was directed to do his preparing and compounding in the "east back room of the Hospital," where shelves and a partition were put up "for a shop."[34]

In the spring of 1755, Roberts notified the Board that he was moving away from Philadelphia and John Morgan, apprentice to John Redman, offered to serve in Roberts' place. With Morgan in attendance, the Board, "having heard a good character of him," hired the future founder of the medical school of the College of Philadelphia, at the same salary as his predecessor. On May 1, 1756, the Board was informed that John Morgan had resigned since

> "he had a prospect of business more advantageous than his present employment."

John Bond, Thomas Bond's nephew, filled the position for two years, but then resigned because of a more "advantageous" prospect and James Ashton Bayard, a student of Thomas Cadwalader, was hired. Intent upon cutting back expenses the Board proposed, as a future policy, to appoint as apothecary "a young student of physic and surgery" without salary. The Board felt that a young student could be convinced of the desirability of serving without salary because of the "advantage" of such an experience. The Board's proposal was not to go into effect, however, until doctors Moore and Shippen each had a chance to recommend a pupil to serve "on the same terms as the others have had. . . ."[35]

After serving slightly less than a year, James Ashton Bayard resigned and one would expect that the announced plan of the Board, to allow doctors Moore and Shippen to recommend one of their pupils, would be put into effect. But, four days after Bayard's resignation, John Moland, on the recommendation of doctors Thomas Bond and John Redman, offered to serve gratis as apothecary for a year. Poor health forced Moland to resign within two weeks and for almost a year the Hospital was without an apothecary.

Because of two other staff resignations, the Hospital found itself without a matron and steward as well as an apothecary. George Weed, from Haddonfied, New Jersey, had previously applied for the position of apothecary, but the Board had not acted favorably on his application. Weed now offered to

> "bring with him his wife and daughter (of about 14 years); he to undertake the care of it as steward and apothecary and his wife to act in the capacity of matron, who with their daughter are to perform such services as that station requires, for all which he proposes the rate of £70 per annum and is willing to contract for four years."

The committee of the Board, sent to Haddonfield to inquire about the Weeds, found that they were well thought of. After an unusually vigorous debate at a Board meeting held on January 7, 1760, Weed and his wife were hired. Leading the opposition to Weed was Israel Pemberton, although the reasons for Pemberton's objections are not recorded. Weed fell ill at that point and it was not until May 14, 1760, that he was feeling well enough to assume his dual responsibilities of apothecary and steward.[36]

Israel Pemberton's objections to Weed may have been based on the suspicion that the latter was a poor apothecary. If so, Pemberton's position was later vindicated. Although George Weed would later advertise his skills in Philadelphia newspapers, in 1767, after noting that Weed was not "so fully qualified as we could wish," the Board consented to the termination of his employment with the Hospital. Weed had resigned in a huff after the Board refused his demand for a salary increase.

Desiring an apothecary "of abilities superior to the last," and unable to find "a fully approved" one who would offer his services, the Board asked Fothergill to choose an apothecary from Great Britain, and send him over. In order to clarify any questions in the minds of prospective candidates, Fothergill was told that the new apothecary needed to be

"so well skilled in the affairs of chemistry as to be able to manage a small laboratory if it should be found necessary."

He would be expected to "do duty in the house as is customary in small hospitals in England," and,

"In order to obviate any fears of having too great employment, he may be informed that the business of dressing . . ."

was to be done by the physicians and pupils of the Hospital. While awaiting help from abroad, the Board employed John Davis as apothecary at £40 per year. Because Davis was not as well qualified as the physicians and the Board wanted—the physicians seem to have a great deal to say about the hiring of apothecaries—and because there was hope that an apothecary could be supplied from England in about a year, Davis agreed to serve for one year and then give up his job after that period on one month's notice.[37]

In the spring of 1768, Robert Slade arrived from Bristol, England, and was hired as steward-apothecary at forty guineas per year. The Managers also consented to pay ten guineas for Slade's passage and to "accommodate him with lodging, diet and washing in the House. . . ." In the Hospital hierarchy, Slade would work, as did previous apothecarie, "under the direction of the physicians." Although John Fothergill and Timothy Bevan did not have the opportunity to meet Slade before his departure for America and, therefore, had been unable to recommend him, the new apothecary had the recommendations of Joseph Fry, Bristol apothecary, and William Logan, cousin of Israel Pemberton. Evidently confident in the new apothecary's credentials, the Board decided to construct a separate two story building, "with all possible dispatch," to serve as a laboratory. Slade did not enjoy his new laboratory for more than a few months before a severe fever ended his service to the Hospital. On July 15, 1769, he was buried in St. Peters Church yard, "his funeral being attended by the Managers, doctors and a number of reputable inhabitants." [38]

Immediately, the Board wrote to John Fothergill and Timothy Bevan in hopes that the two London Quakers could find another Englishman to fill the vacant steward-apothecary position. The Board wanted

"single single person of good character, stability and experience, of middle age and completely capable . . ."

to serve at an annual salary not exceeding £100 Pennsylvania currency and passage money amounting to twelve guineas. The proposed salary was "much beyond what [had] been given at anytime before . . ." because the Hospital had hopes "of being completely supplied." Although Slade's death occurred "at the time of year the Hospital hath the smallest number of patients . . ." the number of patients was steadily increasing and the lack of a steward-apothecary was, to say the least, inconvenient to the Hospital. [39]

In May of 1770, William Smith arrived in Philadelphia bearing letters of recommendation from Fothergill and Bevan as well as a contract between himself and Bevan who had acted on the Hospital's behalf. The Board was very satisfied with Smith's work as steward-apothecary and was, no doubt, unhappy when Smith expressed a desire to leave the Hospital in 1773. Thomas Boulter, assistant apothecary to William Smith, agreed to fill in as apothecary only until a more suitable person could be provided. Boulter served only a couple of months before it was agreed that £70 a year would be paid to an apothecary duly recommended by the physicians. The physicians chose James Hutchinson, nephew to Israel Pemberton, apprentice to Cadwalader Evans and a student at the medical school of the College of Philadelphia.

Because Hutchinson did not also serve as steward, he received some £30 less per year than William Smith. Hutchinson resigned in 1775— he and earlier apothecary John Morgan would later be elected physicians to the Hospital—to be replaced by James Dunlap. Dunlap's qualifications must have been a good deal less impressive than Hutchinson's, as he received only £50 per year. Dunlap, however, proved to be very satisfactory and upon his resignation in the spring of 1776, the Board,

"being well satisfied with his conduct during his attendance agreed to give him a certificate thereof." [40]

During the colonial period the Hospital's apothecaries were the highest salaried members on the staff. They lived in the Hospital, took their meals there and acted as druggist, house physician, and, sometimes, as steward and instructor to apprentices. [41] The eleven apothecaries who served during the colonial period were not a homogenous group. The two Englishmen, Robert Slade and William Smith, earned a considerable salary while John Moland served the Hospital gratis for a year. Two of the apothecaries, John Morgan and James Hutchinson, were obviously ambitious young men on the make, while the likes of George Weed had neither the ambition nor the abilities to handle the job in admirable fashion. But in all, the apothecaries represented the best that the Board could recruit. Although usually not of the same caliber as the physicians, the Pennsylvania Hospital's apothecaries were the elite of the Hospital's salaried staff and, in general, carried out their duties in a responsible manner.

The Matron

Often, during their early years, British voluntary hospitals functioned without a male executive. By default the matron assumed the prerogatives of the chief executive officer. The Pennsylvania Hospital closely emulated the British pattern. Elizabeth Gardner, the first matron, was responsible for the purchasing, keeping the accounts and, with the exception of the apothecary, the direction of the paid staff. Mrs. Gardner's salary included room and board for herself and her two children plus £20 per annum; but so well did this Quaker widow execute her responsibilities that a very pleased Board gave her a £10 per annum raise in 1757. In 1759, Elizabeth Gardner informed the Managers that she was getting married and wished to give up her matron's job. The Board, facing a crisis because of the resignations of the steward and apothecary, persuaded her to remain until the new apothecary-steward, George Weed, and the new matron, Weed's wife Esther, arrived from Haddonfield, New Jersey. In June of 1760, a month after the Weeds had finally arrived, a grateful Board

> "agreed to allow Elizabeth Gardner, late matron, the sum of ten pounds in consideration of her extraordinary services the last six months before she left the Hospital. . . ."[42]

George Weed's wife, Esther, served as matron with the same dedication, although not the authority, of her predecessor. Her husband, in his capacity as steward, took over responsibility for the hospital's financial records and direction of the male employees. The matron did continue to purchase the supplies and give direction to the female staff. On New Year's Day, 1767, Esther Weed caught "a violent cold" and died a few weeks later of an "inflamatory fever." The Board, which was not particularly pleased with George Weed, made it a point to praise the dead matron.[43]

Mary Ball was hired to replace Esther Weed on a trial basis for six months. Her salary was set at £30 per year—Esther Weed's salary had been part of the total of £70 paid George Weed—and, initially at least, she met with Board approval. But by late spring of 1768, the Board had become disenchanted with the matron. When George Weed resigned as steward, Mary Ball took over the management of the Hospital's accounts. Elizabeth Gardner had been equal to the task but, unfortunately, Mary Ball was not. On May 9, 1768, the Board, upset because the fiscal year that ended on May 1 was more expensive than any former year, assigned a committee to investigate ways of reducing expenses. On May 28 the Board's committee reported back

> "that the most effectual means of obtaining the necessary regulation in the economy thereof is that another matron be employed. . . ."

Mary Ball was then paid her full wages and dismissed.[44]

Sarah Harlan, a Quaker, was chosen to replace Mary Ball as matron, at the same salary as her predecessor, but the purchasing and record keeping were placed under the new steward-apothecary, Robert Slade. But like her predecessors, when the occasion arose, Sarah Harlan briefly took over the duties of steward. Sarah Harlan's work pleased the Board a great deal; and, when death ended her service as matron on December 31, 1772, the Board held her funeral at the Hospital. In advertising for a new matron, the Board did not hesitate to extoll the virtues of the recently deceased matron. The Board then turned to a husband and wife team to fill the positions of steward and matron. Sophia and John Saxton were hired after they offered themselves "for three years certain" at £75 per year. The Saxtons had two sons who lived at the Hospital, but the parents paid £15 per year for each child's board and room. The records of the Hospital indicate that the Board had no serious complaint about the Saxtons, but when the Saxtons asked to terminate their contract with the Hospital in 1776, the Managers recorded no word of praise for Sophia Saxton's three years of service.[45]

The Steward

During the eighteenth century, the steward's responsibilities in the British voluntary hospitals were not clearly spelled out.[46] By contrast, in the Pennsylvania Hospital, the steward's responsibilities were clearly delineated. On December 17, 1756, the Hospital was moved from its original site in Judge Kinsey's House to the newly constructed building on Eighth and Pine Streets. The move to the new structure meant a large increase in patients. The next year, realizing that matron Gardner needed help, the Board hired Janathan Norton to

> "take care of the lunaticks, to use his endeavors to oblidge the patients to observe the rules of the House, to assist the matron in the general care of the patients and in marketing, to keep the garden lotts in order and diverse other services now mentioned to him . . ."

at £30 per year.[47]

Although Norton was not called steward—Matthew Taylor, Norton's successor, was the first to officially receive the title—Norton's activities adumbrated those of the later chief administrators of the Hospital.

After unsuccessfully requesting a £20 salary increase per annum, Norton left the Hospital and Jonathan Taylor was hired at the same salary as his predecessor.[48] Although the Hospital now had a steward, matron Elizabeth Gardner continued to be the chief executive of the Hospital until her resignation in 1760. Given the predilection of that day for paying women less than their male counterparts, the fact that both Norton and Taylor were paid the same salary as the matron, indicates Norton and Taylor's subservient position in the eyes of the Managers. Indeed, Norton's request for a salary increase can be seen as a challenge to Mrs. Gardner's position of authority. If the Board had granted the increase it would have been tantamount to recognizing that Norton, rather than Mrs. Gardner, would henceforth be the chief executive officer.

In 1760, with the resignation of Elizabeth Gardner and the hiring of George Weed as steward-apothecary and Esther Weed as matron, the relationship between steward and matron reversed itself with the steward becoming the chief administrative officer, and the matron assuming a subservient position. In part, this was an extension of the marital relationship in which George Weed was the dominant party.[49] Although George Weed, as apothecary, left much to be desired, one gets the feeling—intuitive to be sure—that George Weed, as steward, performed satisfactorily.

Steward-apothecaries Robert Slade and William Smith never allowed the newly developed powers of steward to diminish. Only briefly, when there was no steward, would the matron again assume primary executive responsibilities. Both Slade, who served as steward-apothecary from 1768 to 1769, and William Smith, who served in the same position from 1770 to 1773, were well thought of. But John Saxton, who followed Smith as steward, received no such recorded praises. Perhaps the Board didn't like the fact that Saxton used his indentured servant as a salaried cell keeper. Evidently the servant's salary ended up in Saxton's pockets.[50]

The salaries paid to the Hospital's stewards are difficult to assess, due to the joint nature of the appointments of many of the stewards. How much was alloted for their services as steward, and how much to their services as apothecary? Nevertheless, an examination of stewards' salaries indicates that, by the 1770's, in addition to room and board, the Hospital's steward was paid £45 per year, its matron £30 per year, and its apothecary £70 per year. These wages were higher than those paid in comparable British hospitals.[51]

Cell Keepers

Back in 1750, Quaker John Smith noted the growing problem of lunacy and it was, in part, to meet this social problem that the Pennsylvania Hospital was founded. In the Hospital's first fourteen months, (1752 to 1753) 22 percent of the patients admitted, were lunatics. Obviously, the matron could not handle such potentially violent patients, and so the Hospital hired a male cell keeper. The position of cell keeper seemed to attract a large number of undesirables, but no wonder, when we examine the job! Could any but the less desirable elements of society find attractive the "handling of violent lunatics?"

The turnover in cell keepers, as might be expected, was very high and it was particularly so in the spring and summer of 1752. William Sweeting, then John Baxter, and finally Patrick Motley held the position. Sweeting may have left of his volition, but John Baxter was dismissed in early July, and public notice was given to fill the vacancy. Within five days Patrick Motley was on the job at £20 per year but was warned that if he

> "misbehaves himself the Board resolves to discharge him immediately on such misbehavior. . . ."

Subsequent events justified the Board's uneasiness. Less than two months after being hired, Motley was discharged because he "had been in drink, and very abusive to the matron." Other cell keepers to follow the same path included John McGuire and Charles Bisey.[52]

But for every cell keeper fired, another was soon found to take his place, for the salary of £20 per year and the offer of free board and room was tempting to lower class Philadelphians.[53] The ethnic background of the cell keepers included a strong strain of Celtic stock with such Irish names as Doyle, Finnegan, McGuire and Kelley being represented. Whereas the Quaker affiliations of some of the matrons and stewards were quite evident, no mention is made of any cell keeper being Quaker. Of course, this does not preclude such a possibility. However, the lack of praise from Board members, and the often undesirable actions of the cell keepers, leads me to suspect that the religious affiliations of the cell keepers, if any, were not with the Society of Friends.

Nurses

During the eighteenth century, the traditional view that nurses had little to do with the recovery of the patient was only beginning to give way, and nurses were neither trained nor expected to have much education. Essentially, nurses were more servants than a trained part of the medical team. Lacking in prestige and offering hours of hard, and often distasteful work, nursing positions at hospitals in Great Britain were often difficult to fill. Those nurses who were recruited were drawn from the lower classes and often disreputable. Often they seemed to be indifferent to the welfare of their patients.

Initially, the Pennsylvania Hospital hired maid-nurses to function just as their title indicated. At least two maid-nurses were employed simultaneously until 1754, when, for the first time, the records indicate that the two jobs were separated. Thus the Hospital continued to move towards increased specialization in its personnel, a process that had begun with the hiring of its first apothecary in December of 1752. Newly hired females now found themselves functioning as either nurses or maids, but never, in theory at least, as both. Even though freed from most maid work, nursing in the Pennsylvania Hospital was not overly attractive. The nurse's responsibilities—the records never do spell them out—were probably similar to those of their counterparts elsewhere. They must have included carrying food, tending fires, bathing patients, emptying vessels, handling dressings, quieting disturbances and even burying the dead.[54]

Nurses' salaries at the Pennsylvania Hospital ran between £8 and £20 per year, plus room and board, a somewhat higher sum then paid in Great Britain's provincial hospitals.[55] Although the new building, first occupied in December of 1756, offered clean and well ventilated working conditions, this was not enough to offset the nature of the work—"low and repugnant" according to one European source—and therefore some of the nurses attracted to the Hospital were of the same calibre as most of the cell keepers. Maid-nurse Margaret Sherlock was dismissed in 1754 after frequent complaints over her "disordering herself with strong drink." In 1760, nurse Mary Brown, "having not agreed for sometime past . . ." with the matron and steward, and exhibiting "faulty" conduct, was fired. In 1767, Elizabeth Ball, daughter of matron Mary Ball, was hired as nurse to replace the recently discharged Jane Halfpenny.[56]

But not all the reports on the Hospital's nurses were of a negative nature. Occasionally an exceptional nurse would appear, whose concern for the patients equalled or surpassed that shown by any of the physicians and Managers. In 1755, the Hospital hired Mary Jones, formerly a nurse at St. Thomas's in London, who revealed a charitable bent to her nature when she repeatedly supplied security-burial deposits for a number of the sick-poor, seeking admission. 1757, Mary Jones demanded a raise from £14 to £18, and the Board, no doubt in tribute to her outstanding work, unhesitatingly granted her request.[57] Because of the infrequent mention of nurses in the Hospital's records, other Mary Joneses probably existed but are overlooked, because no records of their activities are extant.

There is no listing of the total number of nurses employed during the colonial period but fragmentary evidence indicates that periodic turnover, although quite high, was not as high as that found among the cell keepers. Nursing salaries, which included room and board, were lowest when nursing was combined with maid work.[58] The number of nurses, at a given time, varied according to the number of patients. After 1754, when maid work and nursing became separate functions, only one nurse was needed. With the occupation of the new building in 1756 and the resulting increase in patients, sometimes as many as two or three nurses were employed. Evidently nurses were assigned to individual floors because, in 1763, the Hospital's records disclose that Jane Moreland was to serve as nurse "for the upper wards."[59] Head nurses were neither needed nor thought of, as direction for the nurses came from the matron.

Maids

In 1754, only one Hospital maid was on the payroll, but by 1759, because of the increased number of patients, three were simultaneously employed. The number of maids at a given time, seemed to bear an inverse relationship to the number of nurses employed. In the 1760's for example, when there were only one or two nurses on the payroll, three maids were employed. During the early 1770's, however, when the number of nurses was increased to three, the number of maids decreased to one or two.[60] Obviously, some of the nurses, during the five years prior to the American Revolution, must have done some maid work, and the maids, during the 1760's, must have helped out with some nursing responsibilities.

As was typical of the cell keepers, the maid positions were subject to constant turnover. Although girls who filled those positions were of lower class background and were probably, in many cases, indentured servants, the number of Irish names, so common among the cell keepers, is not evident among the maids. Salaries for the Hospital's domestics averaged in the neighborhood of £10 per year and probably included room and board. This was a higher salary than paid provincial hospital maids in Great Britain, and about 50 to 70 percent of the salaries earned by nurses at Eighth and Pine.[61]

The matron, steward, apothecary, cell keepers, nurses and maids represented the resident staff of the Hospital, but by no means, incorporated all of the employed personnel. A cook, gardener, and "washer woman" were also on the payroll while periodic visits by carpenters were quite common.[62]

Admissions

Because the purpose of the Pennsylvania Hospital was to cater, in particular, to the industrious sick-poor, nonpaying patients far outnumbered paying patients during the colonial period (see Appendix). There are no extant records on the number of sick-poor who applied, but because funds available to support free beds were limited, only a restricted number of charity patients could be admitted at any one time. In 1774, when the Hospital's income, generated by the capital stock, soared to a record £1,264, there was only enough money to support seventy free beds. By expending current donations, the Hospital could push the number of free patients that it could simultaneously house, to over one hundred;[63] but this meant jeopardizing the long range interests of the Hospital because these contributions were not being added to the capital stock. In short, sometimes the Pennsylvania Hospital accepted more sick-poor patients than, given its financial situation, it should have; but many other sick-poor must have sought admission, only to be turned away.

Once admission regulations had been successfully navigated, the patient was still not assured that he could remain for an extensive period of time. As in the case of British voluntary hospital patients, the sick residents of the Pennsylvania Hospital were to be discharged if, "after a reasonable tryal," their cases were now judged incurable. But in a number of cases when patients were judged incurable and had no place to go, they were allowed, temporarily, to continue their residence at Eighth and Pine. Once, even the ban against contagious diseases was overlooked, when a patient was admitted with smallpox in 1762, and discharged cured a year later.[64]

The total number of Hospital admissions varied from year to year, according to the beds available, and the income generated by the capital stock. Starting with sixty-four patients in 1753—the Hospital year ended on the Saturday preceding the last Monday in April—the yearly admission totals reached a record 538 in 1774. In looking at this upward surge in admissions, two vital explanatory factors must be kept in mind: first, the construction of the new Hospital building at Eighth and Pine which was first occupied, although not completed, in December of 1756; second, the dramatic increases in income, resulting from large increases in the capital stock in 1762 and 1773 (see Appendix).

Just as the total yearly admissions increased dramatically during the colonial period, so too, did the number of patients in the Hospital at any given time (see Appendix). Only nine patients were housed in the Hospital in late May of 1753, but by late April of 1774, one hundred eleven were in residence. Two years later, the residence figure was down to sixty-six, but this was due to the unsettled conditions brought on by the American Revolution.

A comparison of statistics for all patients in residence and all patients admitted, based on figures for the month of April, points out a rather peculiar phenomenon. The residency figures climbed gradually upward to about one hundred patients in 1764, and then leveled off until the decline of 1776. The admission figures, however, show a continued climb after 1765, reaching an all-time peak in 1774.[65] Evidently, the patients admitted to the Hospital in the mid-1760's stayed longer than patients admitted in the late 1760's and early 1770's.

The Pennsylvania Hospital was initially founded to receive the mentally, as well as the physically ill, but this soon led to problems. The mentally ill tended to stay much longer than the physically ill—in some cases for a number of years—and, therefore, ocupied more beds and represented a larger percentage of patients in residence than the initial admission figures indicate. Although no mention is made in the Hospital's records, the possibility that the Hospital could become, primarily, an insane asylum must have worried the Managers. A one-month sampling from the years 1755 to 1776 implicitly reflects the admitting officers' concern over this problem. Only once, in 1762, were enough "lunatics" admitted to approach 50 percent of the total number of patients in residence. After 1762, the percentage of insane admissions seems to have been so regulated as to keep the resident insane figure at about one-third of the total resident figure (see Appendix).[66] Thus, the danger that the Pennsylvania Hospital would become, primarily, an insane asylum was averted during the colonial period.

Paying Patients

After as many sick-poor had been admitted as the Hospital's financial situation could support, the remaining beds and cells were used to accommodate paying patients. During the first decade of the Hospital's existence, approximately 22 percent of the Hospital's sick residents were paying patients. During its second decade, with the Hospital able to support an increased number of free patients, paying patients dropped to only 13 percent of the total.

At the Royal Infirmary of Edinburgh, the only British voluntary hospital to regularly admit paying patients, most of the paying patients were classified as insane. In fact, none of Edinburgh's admitted insane patients were supposed to be charity cases. By contrast, in the Pennsylvania Hospital some of the insane patients were impoverished, and not expected to pay their way. A sampling breakdown for the colonial period shows that insane paying patients at Eighth and Pine never amounted to much more than 50 percent of the total "lunatics" in residence. But of the paying patients, the insane were a disproportionately large percentage. Although the insane may have represented only one-third of the Hospital's resident patients at any given time, probably one-half of those resident patients who paid for, or had others pay for their care, were classified as "lunatics."[67]

During the colonial period the standard charge for paying patients was ten shillings per week. Prior to the construction of the new building at Eighth and Pine Streets, this fee hardly allowed the Hospital to break even. Once the new building was completed, and a large number of patients resided therein, costs per patient took a corresponding dip. In 1755, the cost per patient, on a per diem basis, was slightly in excess of one and one half shillings. By 1765, it had dropped to slightly less than one shilling per diem, and would remain around the one shilling mark for the remainder of the colonial period.[68] By the 1760's, the Hospital was clearing almost three shillings per week on its paying patients. Looked at in another way, for every three paying patients admitted, one more poor patient could be admitted gratis.

Black Patients

Not all paying patients were charged the flat rate of ten shillings per week. Some were charged less simply because they, their relatives or thir masters, could afford no more.[69] In the case of blacks, the Hospital adopted, what seems on the surface, a rather puzzling policy. Some free blacks were admitted as poor patients, on the same basis as whites. Slaves, however, were a different matter. At first all slaves were admitted as paying patients, at the standard rate of ten shillings per week, with the master expected to bear the cost. In 1761, however,

> "it being observed that several Negro slaves have been taken into the House as pay patients at a rate lower than we think can be afforded, it is unanimously agreed that none be hereafter received at less than fifteen shillings per week and as much as the sitting managers shall think the circumstances of the case may require."

In that same year, Cuff, a Negro slave of Dr. Vanliers, who was suffering from "ulcers and carriers," was admitted as a pay patient, at twenty shillings per week. Perhaps the price was too steep for Cuff's master, because Cuff was soon discharged at the request of Vanliers. Later Cuff was readmitted and had a leg amputated, but this time the charge was fifteen shillings per week.[70]

The Managers' explanation, that slaves could no longer be accepted at less than fifteen shillings per week, because the Hospital could not afford it, sounds highly contrived, because the average weekly per patient cost to the Hospital, was well under ten shillings. Despite their statements to the contrary, the Quaker Managers seemed to be raising their fees for the care of slaves as a protest against human bondage. In theory, the master had to pay the extra cost and, therefore, a penalty had been assessed against a supporter of that evil institution. In the case of free Negro George Saunders, a "boy with a round in his arm by an engagement at sea," the Managers further showed their desire to protect blacks from slavery. Nicholas Jones put up security (promised to pay burial expenses) and the Board, wary of the motives behind Jones' generosity, made careful notice that

> "care must be taken on his [Saunders'] discharge that N. Jones takes no advantage of him for his entertainment here."[71]

It might be argued that increasing the Hospital's charge for slaves hurt the individual slaves more than it hindered the institution of slavery. Masters would now hesitate to send their sick and injured slaves to the Hospital because the cost was too steep. On the other hand, the Managers probably felt that by charging more for slaves, they were at least giving vent to their distaste for America's "peculiar institution." Although a small gesture, the action of the Managers takes on more meaning when viewed against the backdrop of rising Quaker antipathy to slavery.[72]

Venereal Patients

Paying patients suffering from venereal disease represented a particular conundrum. Obviously the "wages of sin," venereal disease could not be classified in the same category as "dropsy" or "scorbutick ulcers" or "consumption." If the Managers turned away those afflicted with venereal disease, their Christian charity would be suspect. But equal treatment of venereal and non-venereal patients could be interpreted as a passive stand on a significant moral issue.

From the beginning, impoverished sufferers of all non-contagious disease (including venereal) were received gratis. Thus in 1759, Thomas Wilkins, a poor sailor "with venereal disorder," was admitted. Wilkins was one of the first venereal patients, but up until 1762, venereal patients were not very numerous. On September 22, 1762, however, six female venereal cases were admitted and Redmund Cunningham, who may have been exercising a laudable interest in his employees' welfare, agreed to pay "ten shillings per week for each." Faced with the possibility of being further inundated by venereal patients, the Board gave deep thought to the situation, and decided, the following year, that no venereal patients were to be admitted unless "in apparent danger of perishing and cannot be accommodated elsewhere."[73] Despite these stipulations, by 1767 almost 9 percent of the in-patients treated were suffering from venereal disease. In February of 1768, the Managers, evidently feeling that those Philadelphians who could afford to, ought to pay for their transgressions,

> "resolved that all patients hereafter received on pay infected with venereal disease, shall pay at least fifteen shillings a week for their board and nursing."[74]

The singling out of venereal paying patients for extra fees was not a uniquely American development. Venereal patients in some of Great Britain's hospitals were also singled out and forced to pay extra fees.

The impact of the rate increase on venereal paying patients is difficult to assess. By 1769, venereal patients of both paying and non-paying categories, represented about 11 percent of the resident patients; this was a 3 percent increase over the 1767 figure. [75] But since the records do not differentiate between paying and non-paying venereal patients, we can not automatically assume that the number of the latter increased because of the increase in the weekly rate.

Out-Patients

Besides treating some 6,581 in-patients during the colonial period, the Hospital simultaneously ran an out-patient department.[76] Unfortunately, we have only a few fragmentary pieces of evidence concerning out-patient care. In January of 1754, there were four out-patients, while in February of the following year three out-patients were treated. Fragmentary reports in the succeeding years indicate that monthly recorded high for out-patients during the colonial period was reached in June of 1774, when twenty-eight were treated. In May of 1775, the Board directed the sitting managers

> "to report the number of out-patients monthly admitted, it appearing that for sometime past, they had considerably increased."

The annual report of the next year indicated that some one hundred ninety-eight out-patients were treated in a twelve month period.[77]

Open Vistas

Physical accommodations at the Pennsylvania Hospital were thought by many to compare very favorably with accommodations in British and European hospitals. But it wasn't only the building that was of particular significance on this account. Increasingly, hospital reformers were calling for wide open spaces around their institutions, which could supply fresh "healing" breezes and insulate the Hospital from the spread of epidemics and fire. In 1752, the Board asked the Proprietor—to no avail to be sure—for part of a square on the south side of Mulberry, between Ninth and Tenth Streets. This plot seemed attractive as a hospital site because

"in all probability there will be a conveniency of an open air for many years. . . ."[78]

No doubt, part of the attraction of the eventual site on Eighth and Pine Streets was the same probability of "open air."

The Hospital was not content to occupy only part of the square bordered by Spruce, Pine, Eighth and Ninth Streets. In 1767, the remainder of that square was acquired through the benevolence of the Proprietor (see chapter II). Thanks to another donation by the Penns, the purchase of two lots for £500, and plot trading with the Philadelphia Almshouse, by 1769 the Hospital controlled most of the block directly to its west. By 1776, the Hospital had purchased all but a small strip along Pine Street of the block directly to the east. The blocks to the south and north seemed, for the time being at least, to offer no threat to the bucolic setting of the Hospital and no serious attempt was made to purchase these properties.[79]

Patient Care

It is difficult to get a clear picture of actual conditions inside the Hospital's "large and neat brick building." As stipulated by the Hospital's charter, a committee of the colonial legislature made annual visits and always seemed to be very satisfied with what it found. In 1775, however, no record of the legislature's committee visiting the Hospital is extant. Perhaps, given the unrest of the times, the legislators had more important duties to occupy their time. Nevertheless, we do have the observations of a forign visitor to fill us in on what the representatives of the Pennsylvania legislature would have seen. Dr. Robert Honyman, a Scotsman and son of a Presbyterian minister, visited the Hospital on March 7, 1775, and complained that he

"was by no means pleased with the appearance of the inside [of the Hospital] and the accommodations and looks of the patients."

But the available evidence does not support this supposition. The attending Managers, a two-man committee of the Board appointed for a one month period, with responsibility for admissions, and the overall direction of the Hospital, only two weeks prior to Honyman's visit, reported that the Hospital was clean, and the patients were well taken care of. The attending Managers' reports for March and April are not extant, but May's report was equally laudatory except that some of the patients were "in want of necessary clothing . . ."

Perhaps a more objective observer was John Adams who had visited the Hospital during the previous year. Although Adams found the sick wards to be "a dreadful scene of human wretchedness," he made no mention of specific shortcomings of the Hospital, and was probably indirectly praising that institution, when he noted that Boston was superior to Philadelphia, except in its "Markett, and in charitable Foundations."[81] But then John Adams had never visited other hospitals—at this time the Pennsylvania Hospital was the only institution of its type in the thirteen colonies[82] and John Adams had yet to cross the Atlantic—and, therefore, unlike Dr. Honyman, he had no way of comparing the Pennsylvania Hospital with other institutions of its type.

Contradiction of Dr. Honyman's observations on conditions in the Pennsylvania Hospital is not restricted to eighteenth century observers. Carl Bridenbaugh, in *Rebels and Gentlemen*, states that nowhere

"in the western world were such comfortable accommodations and enlightened care provided for the mentally ill . . ."

The care given to the occupants of the sick wards received almost equal praise in Bridenbaugh's lyrical rendition of the Quaker city *"In The Age of Franklin."* One canont help but suspect, however, that Professor Bridenbaugh, intent on having the Hospital play a positive role in the unfolding success story of colonial Philadelphia, brushed aside, too quickly, Honyman's criticism. While Professor Bridenbaugh is correct in saying that most visitors to the Hospital came away with a positive impression, one wonders how many of these "visitors" had seen other hospitals.[83] In short, a precise declaration concerning overall conditions in the Hospital during colonial times is impossible due to conflicting observations and the paucity of other evidence. This does not preclude, however, some general observations on specific areas of Hospital life.

In Europe, during the second half of the eighteenth century, the introduction of iron beds and the easy-to-wash cotton blanket helped make hospital beds less hospitable to lice and other vermin. During the colonial period some iron beds were in use in the Pennsylvania Hospital, but no mention is made of cotton bed clothing. Linen of Oznaburg or Russian variety was purchased and, because of the constant use by the Hospital of a washerwoman, one can suppose that bed linens were washed often.[84] Indeed, if no attempt was made to keep up to certain standards, middle class paying patients would not have sought admission nor would relatives of those same patients been inclined to contribute to the Hospital's capital stock.

The Insane

The conditions under which the insane lived were of particular concern to the Board and the physicians. Many insane patients were violent and some "lunatics" had to be kept in the cells directly below the men's ward. The individual cells had plank floors "arched below to prevent dampness, and preclude association with rats." Since wood fires in the cells were impossible, the insane must have been miserably damp and cold during the winter months, but then the insane were said to be insensitive to cold. In 1762, the Managers ordered a platform built over the outside wall of the cells, to protect the cells from water dripping from the eaves of the roof, but the platform did little to blunt the harsh winter cold. Iron bars covered the windows of the cells, while iron chains were attached to the feet and hands of the most violent patients.[85]

Despite efforts to keep the insane from bothering their fellow patients, disturbances were not uncommon and escapes were numerous. In 1754, for example, Thomas Hutchinson had to be discharged because

"the patients suffer so much by his noise, particularly Mary Jefferson whose life is in danger for want of rest. . . ."

In 1758, Jane Hughes became so violent that she damaged her cell! Even the cells' bars could not hold back insane patients, Jonathan Jones and Charles Jenkins. By forcing apart the iron bars, Jones and Jenkins escaped from their respective cells on at least seven separate occasions, only to be brought back. In 1758, faced with the repeated successful escapes of Jones and Jenkins, the Board decided that a blacksmith be called in to "make their [iron bars] stronger and more secure." But even this measure did not seem to be enough, as a year later Jenkins escaped again "by breaking out the iron bars over the cell door." Jenkins continued to plague the Hospital with further escapes, but none of Jenkin's breakouts approached the sophisticated method used by Jacob Ashton, who escaped

"by boring through the door of the cell and forcing out the staples of the iron bolts."

Escapes by insane patients continued to plague the Hospital, with the monthly high of seven "elopments" recorded for August of 1773. Sometimes, discontent among the insane could take a more somber form, as in April of 1765, when a distraught patient hanged himself.[86]

To Philadelphians, the insane were objects of curiosity, to be viewed with the same interest as zoo animals, and the inmates at Eighth and Pine sometimes performed for the curious and sadistic public in a rather bizarre fashion. In 1759, for example, insane patient Martin Higgins

"as many others do without leave [went] through the House ot the top and there carelessly and imprudently running about fell from thence to the ground and was so much bruised and hurt that his recovery was doubtful [and] was immediately brought into the House and still remains."

In another case, former sailor Thomas Perrine was admitted in 1765, but soon escaped from his basement cell and raced through the Hospital until he found refuge in the cupola, from where he successfully resisted all efforts to dislodge him. Finally, Hospital authorities abandoned their attempts to get him down and sent up bedding and food. Noted for his long nails and matted beard and hair, from his perch, Perrin must have loomed like some malevolent bird-spirit to onlookers from below. Seemingly insensitive to cold weather, Perrin continued to occupy the cupola until his death in 1774.

Because the public felt free to wander through the Hospital to view the objects of their interest, in 1760, the Managers proposed a

"suitable palisade fence . . . should be erected in order to prevent the disturbance which is given to the lunatics confined in their cells by the great numbers of people who frequently resort and converse with them."

The fence, however, nas not enough to keep out the curious and sadistic. In 1763, a "hatch door" was constructed, with an inscription on it to

"notify that such persons who came out of curiousity to view the House should pay a sum of money, a grout at least [a grout was equal to four pence] for admittance, the great crowds who resort here of late, giving trouble and disturbance."[87]

The Managers again had demonstrated their resourcefulness by turning an annoying problem into an economic asset. But, at what cost to the peace and tranquility of the insane?

The Daily Routine

Given the veneration for the "work ethic" among eighteenth century Philadelphians, it is not surprising that patients who were physically able, were put to work. In 1754, for example, Managers Isaac Jones and Evan Morgan agreed to provide some spinning wheels, wool and flax for the use of patients. In a few cases, the Hospital felt obliged to make the work instructional, so that patients with permanent disabilities would be prepared to support themselves, after being discharged from the Hospital. In 1760, after a ten-year-old blind child had been a patient for some time, the Hospital inserted an ad in the *Pennsylvania Gazette* in order to find someone who would

"undertake to instruct her in such business as she may be capable of, to enable her to make a living. . . ."[88]

The diet of the Hospital's patients seems to have been reasonably varied. Few actual menues for the colonial period are extant, but purchasing records and scattered statements support the above generalization. Purchases of beef, veal, pork, mutton, fowl, oysters, butter, cheese, milk, coffee, tea and rum indicate a well balanced diet by the standards of the day. Again, the food had to be up to certain standards, to satisfy paying patients and their families. Just as in British hospitals, special diets were prescribed for certain illnesses. Initially, paying patients may have been better fed than non-paying patients, but in 1768, the Managers resolved that paying patients receive the same diets as the rest.

Lowering food costs was never far from the mind of the Board. In 1759, a committee was set up to regulate the diet of the patients "in order as far as practicable, to lessen the expenses of housekeeping." And yet, the interests of the patients were not overlooked in order to save a few pounds. Improvement in their diet was constantly being considered, and in 1759 and in 1767 new diets were introduced "for the benefit of the patients."[89]

A typical day for a patient at the Hospital is difficult to describe, because no actual details are extant. Beds for the physically ill were lined up along the two long walls of the two wards. There is no indication that curtains were hung around each bed, but consideration of privacy and warmth should have prescribed this practice. Franklin stoves, were, no doubt, used to warm most of the Hospital, but the cells of the insane continued to receive little direct heat throughout the eighteenth century. The patient's day must have been regulated by the sun, causing breakfast to be served early. Nurses and maids then made their way among the patients, emptying bed pans and urine bottles, making beds, sweeping the floor and attending to the numerous other chores that fell their lot. Those patients who could do so, aided in making their less fortunate roommates as comfortable as possible. On two days of the week two doctors, with apprentices in tow, would move slowly through the wards, dressing wounds, prescribing drugs, and offering clinical observations to their eager entourage. About noon, lunch was served. The afternoon found the patients receiving visitors or simply staring vacuously into space. For literate patients, Bibles and other religious tracts were available. Many patients, however, were illiterate and could not resort to reading, to temper the monotony of hospital life. The evening meal was served early and then it was lights out.[90]

Because not all patients behaved in an orderly fashion, the rather dull routine of the Hospital day was occasionally interrupted. By 1762, patient misconduct—exclusive of the insane patients, who have already been mentioned—led the Board to transcribe

> "a sufficient number of the rules of conduct to be observed by the patients to be hung up in the several wards."

But no wonder there was a need for strict rules, when it is considered that, on a couple of occasions, jailed criminals were admitted to the Hospital as paying patients.[91]

Looking at the Record

In the final analysis, pragmatic America judges its institutions by the results achieved. Therefore the question, "How well were the patients of the Pennsylvania Hospital treated during the colonial period?" can best be answered by looking at the record. The assumption is that good care kept patients alive and poor care left them dead. But to merely list the number of patients who were cured, and the number who died in the Pennsylvania Hospital, is not enough. To give real meaning to mortality statistics, a reference group is necessary for comparative purposes, and the logical reference group is the British voluntary and Royal hospitals.

It has generally been assumed that the death rate at the Pennsylvania Hospital was considerably lower than at hospitals across the Atlantic. According to one historian, the Pennsylvania Hospital's mortality rate, prior to the American Revolution, was "half that of general hospital's abroad." Another scholar writes that the death rate at Eighth and Pine, for the same period, was "but a fraction of that in London and Paris hospitals." The facts, however, tell quite a different story.[92]

Recent research has shown that the commonly accepted belief, that a high mortality rate characterized eighteenth century British hospitals, is in error. The available evidence now points to a mortality rate that ranged from 6 to 13 percent of admitted patients.[93] The Pennsylvania Hospital's mortality rate during the colonial period, was 12 percent, which was on the high side of the British average.[94] Of course it can be argued that, unlike British hospitals, the Pennsylvania Hospital housed the insane, who stayed longer, and therefore had a higher mortality rate, than the somatically ill. But random sampling of the resident insane reveals a mortality rate quite similar to the other patients.[95]

The similarity in mortality statistics, is partly explained by the similarity in medical treatment. The physicians at Eighth and Pine had been directed to keep a diagnostic record of each patient's case, and the resulting therapy prescribed.[96] Unfortunately, the physicians' records for the eighteenth century have been lost. Nevertheless, given the academic training of most of the Hospital's physicians, it is safe to deduce that the same bleeding, purging, and sweating that was dispensed as therapy, at the medical centers on the European continent and in Great Britain, was practiced at the Pennsylvania Hospital. Historian Daniel Boorstin's claim, that the American patient had an advantage over his European counterpart, because American practitioners were not as bogged down "with so much learned error,"[97] probably had little relevance to conditions in the Pennsylvania Hospital, because here, the patient was ministered to on the basis of principles believed to be medically sound in London, Edinburgh and Leyden.

Chapter 4

The Crisis Years, 1775-1783

IN MID-APRIL OF 1775, the pastoral calm of the countryside near Boston, was broken by the sharp reports of musket fire. The resulting skirmishes at Lexington and Concord marked the beginning of a new era in American history. As wars go, the American Revolution was not a particularly bloody, or destructive affair. Nevertheless, the resulting turmoil and confusion, inherent in all wars, had a great impact on Philadelphia, in general, and on the Pennsylvania Hospital, in particular.

During the unsettled years of the Revolution, the Hospital received a vigorous buffeting, which threatened not only the success, but the very existence of that institution. In 1774, the Hospital's productive capital stock exceeded £20,000; by 1783, it was down to less than one half that figure. The average number of resident patients, after running well over one hundred in the decade prior to the Revolution, dropped to less than forty, by 1783. Even more alarming was the decline in the number of resident poor patients, which dropped precipitously, from about ninety to twelve, over the same period (see Appendix). All of the available indices reported the same general picture of decline. The war experience, which was so unsettling for Philadelphia, was disastrous for the Pennsylvania Hospital.

Prior to the American Revolution, the fact that the Board of Managers was a predominantly Quaker body did little harm and, indeed, enhanced the reputation of the Hospital in some quarters. Although hostility between Thomas Penn and some Pennsylvania Quakers caused the Proprietor's initial reluctance to grant the Hospital his blessings, the financial support by Philadelphians of all creeds, and by overseas Quakers, more than balanced Penn's negative reaction. The American Revolution, however, created questions in the minds of many Pennsylvanians concerning their Quaker neighbors. Because Friends generally were either neutral or passive loyalists, the revolutionary government of Pennsylvania, and individual rebels, looked upon Quakers as spies and informers. Public hostility took the form of double taxation, imprisonment, and even exile.

To add to their problems, Quakers usually were unwilling to engage in war profiteering, or in taking "what advantage they could find of the currency situation." Unable to avoid the pitfalls of non-involvement, and unwilling to take commercial advantage of a fluid situation, many Quakers "felt the pinch on their private fortunes."[1]

In short, Philadelphians, hard pressed because of the unsettled times, and suspicious of the Pennsylvania Hospital because of its Quaker connections, were less willing than in previous years, to open up their purses. The Managers of the Pennsylvania Hospital could not offset the decline in subscriptions, with increased personal contributions, because their own financial situations had deteriorated. From 1770 to 1776, Hospital contributions and legacies combined to average almost £820 per year. For the years 1777 to 1782, however, contributions and legacies combined to average only about £178 per year.[2]

The Board of Managers

During the Revolution, the Hospital continued to be directed by a predominantly Quaker Board of Managers. Of the thirty-three men serving on the Board from 1775 to 1783, twenty-one of them (64 percent) were of the Friendly Persuasion. Moreover, eight out of the eleven Managers who served four years or more during the Revolution, were Quakers. Of the three presidents of the Board, John Reynell and Samuel Rhoads have already been spoken of, concerning their Quaker connections while the third, Peter Reeve, was a birthright Quaker, who had been read out of the Philadelphia Monthly Meeting in 1772. The two treasurers during this period were also Quakers.[3] Moreover, even though the "King of the Quakers," Israel Pemberton, would die in 1779, and other influential Quakers, such as James Pemberton, Samuel Rhoads and John Reynell would resign from the Board during the Revolution, a new generation of Quakers stepped forward to fill the void. The American Revolution witnessed the decline of the "old guard," which had been with the Hospital from its inception, but not at the cost of Quaker hegemony.

Although "neutral" during the Revolution, not all of the Quaker Managers had remained politically passive in the immediate prewar period. Some felt that Americans were justified in protesting new taxes and other restrictive regulations, passed by Parliament. Israel Pemberton opposed the Stamp Act, while John Reynell led the Non-Importation Association against the Townshend Acts. Samuel Rhoads represented Pennsylvania at the First Continental Congress which met in Carpenters' Hall on September 4, 1774. Nevertheless, the

> "number of Friends concerned in radical measures . . . was not large and consisted mostly of youths."[4]

In 1775, the Philadelphia Yearly Meeting warned that Quakers entering into martial engagements would be read out of Meeting. The Pennsylvania Assembly reacted by laying a fine of two pounds, ten shillings, on those who refused military service. Pennsylvania Friends responded by objecting to the growing sentiment for independence, in a paper signed by John Pemberton, Israel's brother. Despite Quaker entreaties to the contrary, independence was declared, and Pennsylvania Whigs wrote a new constitution for the state, and by this act, destroyed William Penn's charter, thought by Israel Pemberton, to be the bulwark of Quaker liberty. From this point on, Philadelphia's Quakers withdrew into themselves and became, in John Adams' words, "a kind of neutral tribe . . .."[5] Non-Quaker Board members joined their Quaker colleagues in remaining aloof from participation in the Revolution.

Neutrality towards the Revolution should not be taken as disinterest in public affairs. The Managers of the Hospital watched anxiously, as one political event led to another, in the deepening crises that inexorably brought serious turmoil to the Quaker City, and to the Hospital at Eighth and Pine. To keep open the Hospital in order to continue to render service to the community in those trying times, was the goal that the Managers kept before them. That the Hospital emerged from the American Revolution seriously weakened, but still alive, is comment enough on the tenacity of the Board during those "crisis years."

The Initial Impact of the Revolution

The first mention of repercussions from the Revolution occurred in late June of 1775, when the Managers noted that "the present state of public affairs will not permit . . ." the importation of more drugs. In July of 1776, a few wounded soldiers were admitted, bringing the impact of the war closer to Eighth and Pine. Meanwhile, the number of resident patients had begun to decline in the late winter and early spring of 1776. By June of 1776, there were only fifty-six patients in the Hospital, a figure that represented about 50 percent of capacity. In November of 1776, William Smith, provost of the College of Philadelphia, offered to pay off a mortgage, held by the Hospital, in part at least in "current money." The Managers hedged on the proposal because they did not want to receive depreciating paper currency. Up to this point (November, 1776), except for the developments cited above, the war had not yet left a great mark on the Hospital.[6]

On December 5, 1776, the Council of Safety (the executive branch of the newly created state of government of Pennsylvania) resolved that the Pennsylvania Hospital "be taken up and employed for the sick troops of the Continental Army. . . ." On that same day, fifty soldiers were admitted as patients. During January, twenty-nine more soldiers, including nineteen Hessians, captured by Washington at Trenton, were admitted. During that month, twenty-two of the soldiers residing in the Hospital died. By the end of February, there were fifty-five soldiers and only thirty-seven civilian patients residing in the Hospital. Thomas Bond had, by this time, placed his services at the disposal of the revolutionaries and, being responsible for the injured and sick military personnel in the Hospital—a few sailors had also been admitted—promised to pay for medicines that he used in healing his military patients.

Although the Hospital was paid for "nursing and curing" the sick soldiers, this additional income (about £194) was not enough to keep the Hospital out of financial trouble. By May, the inflation that would plague Philadelphia throughout most of the war, forced the Hospital to increase its charge for paying patients, from ten to fifteen shillings per week. Two months later, the Managers decided to pay off Hospital bills in the already depreciating Continental currency. Given Quaker reluctance to use revolutionary money, one gets the picture of the desperate plight of the Board as it abandoned Quaker discipline for practical expedients, to save the Hospital.[7]

British Occupation

By the late spring of 1777, most of the Continental soldiers had left the Hospital, but respite from military patients was very brief. In late August, General Howe landed some fourteen thousand British soldiers at the head of the Chesapeake Bay, some fifty miles from Philadelphia. Marching north and east to the Brandywine Creek, Howe found rebel forces occupying the east bank because Washington was unwilling to give up Philadelphia, without a fight. After a flanking maneuver, and a strong drive against the center of the rebel lines at Chadd's Ford, General Howe's forces scored a victory at the Battle of the Brandywine, and Washington hurriedly retreated towards Philadelphia. Howe turned northward and made a feint towards Washington's right flank, which caused the Virginian to move his forces westward, as a counter measure. The road to Philadelphia now lay open, and the British entered the Quaker City on September 26. Eight days later, Washington's attempt to drive the British forces from Philadelphia, was frustrated at the Battle of Germantown.

Although Howe was able to turn back rebel attempts to first defend, and then retake, Philadelphia, he was unable to destroy the rebel army, or to dislodge it from positions near the Quaker City. While southeastern Pennsylvania produced numerous neutrals, and some supporters of the crown, Howe's reception in Philadelphia was not particularly enthusiastic, and only slightly more than three hundred Tory troops were recruited from the area. Moreover, Howe's expedition against Philadelphia abandoned Burgoyne to humiliation and final defeat at Saratoga, in upstate New York. Although Howe had captured the rebel capital, Congress escaped westward to York, and in May of 1778, realizing the failure of his Philadelphia expedition, Howe resigned and was replaced by General Henry Clinton.

On September 26, 1777, with

> "Part of the British Army, under the command of Sir William Howe arriving in the city, . . . a great number of sick and wounded soldiers (without previous notice given, or application to the Managers) were brought into the Hospital. . . ."

These sick and wounded British soldiers crowded the wards, "incommoding" the civilian patients "and rendering it impracticable to pursue the former good order of the House." By October, the Managers were willing to admit that treatment of Hospital patients had considerably declined. The same admission was repeated the following month, leaving no doubt that the war had brought on a serious deterioration of conditions in the Pennsylvania Hospital. The British compounded the Hospital's difficulties, when they promptly outlawed all payments in Revolutionary currency. With their backs to the wall, the Managers borrowed one hundred pounds, in specie, from fellow Board member Jacob Shoemaker, in order to keep the Hospital functioning.[8]

By January of 1778, there remained in the Hospital, only twenty-nine civilian patients. Except for Thomas Bond, the doctors seemed too busy with other duties to make their scheduled rounds. The steward, upon instruction from the Board, introduced a new diet, that was less expensive to the Hospital, but was also less nourishing to the patients. In desperation, a committee of the Board drew up a memorial to General Howe

"representing the present distressed situation of the Hospital and requesting relief. . . ."

There is no record that Howe responded positively to the plea, although, after a similar request from the Almshouse, he sanctioned the collection of contributions. The same committee was then requested to meet with Dr. Morris, the Inspector General of the British hospitals, to complain of

"the loss in blankets, medicine and hay that the institution has sustained by the admission of the sick and wounded soldiers of their [British] army."

Whether the committee met with Dr. Morris is unclear, but there is no doubt that the British never reimbursed the Hospital for its losses. Another loan of specie, some four hundred pounds, this time, kept the Hospital going until the British evacuated Philadelphia, in June of 1778.[9]

The bad news of Saratoga, and the impending French involvement, caused a change in British military plans for 1778. On March 21, secret instructions were signed by George III, ordering the evacuation of Philadelphia. By June 18, the British army, accompanied by three thousand Tories, was on its way, by both land and sea, to New York. Never again would Philadelphia hear British boots marching on her cobbled streets, nor see the masts of the British fleet, projecting above the houses on Water Street.

The war continued in other sections of the thirteen colonies, however, and the attendant suspicions, shortages, and currency inflation, which are sometimes more disruptive than actual fighting, served to prevent Philadelphia from returning to pre-war normality. Perhaps Scharf and Wescott put it best by stating that

Philadelphia . . . suffered cruelly from the Revolution. Her trade had been prostrated; many of her wealthy citizens had been reduced to want and others driven into exile; her industrial, educational, and social development had been interrupted and set back many years . . ."[10]

Specific Problems and Solutions

The period of British occupation had been particularly difficult for the Hospital because four of the Managers were not in Philadelphia to give counsel. Only fifteen days before Howe's capture of the city, twenty Pennsylvanians — seventeen were Quakers — were taken under guard, to Winchester, Virginia. The rationale for this forced exile was the supposed Tory sympathies of the twenty prisoners. Among the exiles were Managers Israel and James Pemberton, Thomas Wharton, and Edward Pennington. For almost eight months the four Quaker Managers were kept in exile, suffering from poor health. In January, an epidemic of some proportion struck Winchester, and the physical condition of all the exiles was further impaired. Israel Pemberton, once the strong and aggressive leader of the Board, was now "a poor weak old man . . ." while Manager Edward Pennington had become insane. Finally the Council of Safety of Pennsylvania decided to release the prisoners, and the eighteen who still survived—two had died in Winchester—reached Philadelphia on April 29, after some eight months of exile. The return of the exiles brought new life to the Hospital, just as it brought new vigor to Quaker Meetings in Philadelphia. This new vigor can be seen in the bold demands made to the Inspector General of the British hospitals, and in the initial refusal made in the spring of 1779, to accommodate wounded and sick soldiers of the Continental army."[11]

To meet some of its more specific problems during 1778, the Board searched for solutions not dependent on aid from the British or the Revolutionary government. In August of 1778, "in consideration of the present high price of milk," three cows were purchased. In December of the same year, the Board, "taking into consideration the urgent want of blankets, . . ." appointed a committee to procure an immediate supply. Nevertheless, despite renewed activity on the part of the Board, the Hospital continued to face difficulties, and the Board, in order to cut back costs, even considered "discharging" the steward and matron.[12]

With the reoccupation of Philadelphia by Washington's forces in June of 1778, a slow shift in Quaker sentiment towards the American revolutionaries can be noted, and this change in attitude would affect the Pennsylvania Hospital. Quaker ill feelings toward the revolutionaries, magnified by the exile of the seventeen Quakers to Virginia, "were effectually checked" by the behavior of the British soldiery, in and around Philadelphia, during the disastrous winter of 1777–1778. The revelry into which some young Friends were drawn, and a disregard for property rights by the British, particularly incensed the Quakers. Moreover, the return of the exiles, and the impending British evacuation of Philadelphia, caused many Friends to reconsider their loyalties. Although Pennsylvania Quakers refused to join in public thanksgiving for the American victory at Yorktown in 1781, the Quaker community was already showing signs of acquiescence in a "fait accompli."[13]

In July of 1778, the Hospital agreed to rent its "Elaboratory", to be used for the preparing and compounding of medicines, for the use of the military hospitals of the Continental Army. The Elaboratory was a two story building, detached from the Hospital and used previously by the Hospital's apothecary, for mixing drugs. Two months later, Thomas Bond, Jr., son of the Hospital's founder, and Adjutant General of the Continental Hospital, noting the available space in the Pennsylvania Hospital (there were only thirty-five patients), applied to the Managers for admission of large numbers of Continental soldiers

> "under the direction and management of their [Continental] physicians and surgeons."

The Board objected to Bond's proposal, but did agree to admit Continental soldiers, if certain conditions could be met. The main condition was, that the soldiers be placed under the same regulations as civilian patients. The Board's demand seems to have displeased the Adjutant General, but in March of the following year, Thomas Bond, Jr., made another request to use the facilities of the main Hospital building, only to be turned down by the Board. But Bond was a persistant man and, after complaining that all other facilities were overcrowded, stated that the soldiers would be placed under the care of the Hospital's steward, although a military surgeon would "prescribe to them." Moreover, Thomas Bond, Jr., added that he would be in Philadelphia, and would do everything in his power, to restrain the soldiers from committing damage and behaving badly. Bond also promised to remove all of the soldiers from the Hospital within six weeks.

Evidently convinced by Bond's pleas and wishing, perhaps, to establish better relations with the revolutionary government, the Board agreed to admit the soldiers. The Hospital's new patients were assigned the lower ward and the long garret on the top floor. The Managers reminded Bond that the Hospital expected a reasonable compensation, and that no soldier with "infectuous distemper" could be admitted. By April 26, forty sick and injured Continental soldiers were housed in the Hospital's main building. The soldiers' stay was brief, and the Hospital received £137 from Bond, for the use of its facilities.[14]

The willingness of the Board to cooperate with the Continental army coincided, to the month, with the death of Israel Pemberton. The "King of the Quakers," physically weakened by his recent exile to Virginia, contracted a fever in mid-April, 1779, and died within a week. The dominant figure on the Board of Managers, Pemberton had strongly disapproved of the colonial independence movement. It was self-evident, that as long as Pemberton lived, the Board could not fully cooperate with the Continental Army, or the rebel controlled state government. With Pemberton gone, the other Managers, less uncompromising than their dead colleague, were now free to reach some sort of accommodation with the Continental Army, and the Pennsylvania Assembly.[15]

By September of 1779, accommodation seemed to be working, as a committee representing the Assembly, was sympathetically examining the Hospital's plight. In January of the following year, a petition from the Hospital was delivered to the Assembly, asking for funds from the public treasury. In the memorial to the Assembly, the Board noted that the act of making paper currency legal tender, was a primary cause of the Hospital's financial hardships. Back in December of 1776, some members of Congress believed that Philadelphia's Quakers had determined to refuse Continental paper money. General Putnam, then in command of Philadelphia, issued a severe order against anyone who would not accept paper money. Soon after, the Pennsylvania Assembly declared all State and Continental paper money, to be legal tender. This meant that the Hospital had to accept depreciated paper currency from debtors, who had taken out loans from the Hospital. Quite simply, the Hospital was caught in the bind that all creditor institutions face during inflation; the Hospital was being paid in cheap money, for dear money lent. Some debtors even tried to pay off their loans ahead of time, with depreciated currency, but in these cases the Hospital did have the legal right to refuse.

The memorial went on to complain of

> "the continued depreciation of currency which the treasurer is from time to time oblidged to receive for interest of the capital stock or for rents and the consequent exorbitant charges of housekeeping."

The memorial listed the previous grants from the colonial Assembly "amounting together to five thousand pounds"—evidently some smaller grants were not considered significant enough to mention—which was

> "an inconsiderable sum compared with the liberal benefactions of individuals and the grant of the British Parliament. . . ."

The memorial closed with a request for financial aid from the Assembly. The Assembly responded with a grant of £10,000, but in depreciated Continental currency, which was probably worth about £164 in prewar Pennsylvania currency. To make matters worse, the Assembly looked on this grant as a loan.[16]

The Assembly did grant the Hospital, unclaimed prize money gained from the seizure of British vessels, by certain ships of the Continental Navy. Payments to the Hospital, however, did not begin until May of 1782, and did not amount to much until after the war. Fines paid to the Assembly by individual members of that body, continued to be donated to the Hospital, but never represented a significant amount.[17]

By April of 1783, a troubled Board was directing yet another plea to the Assembly for aid. Back in 1780, when a similar plea for help was addressed to the Assembly, the Hospital was in debt "upwards of £1,100 in specie", and the capital stock had lost, since the beginning of the war, "about eight thousand pounds like money by the receipt of depreciated currency." It was obvious that the Assembly loan of 1780 had done little to improve the Hospital's financial situation. By 1783, some creditors were still awaiting payment for goods, purchased by the Hospital in 1776! The Assembly, its funds exhausted by war, was in no position to grant further succor to the Hospital, but did change the "loan" of 1780 into a clear "grant" to the Hospital.[18]

The Passing of the Old Guard

The Board that sent the appeal to the Assembly in 1783 was not the same body that demanded compensation from the British in 1777 for the loss of "blankets, medicine and hay." Gone were the imposing figures of Israel Pemberton and the other Quaker grandees, responsible for the founding and early success of the Hospital. James Pemberton and John Reynell resigned from the Board in 1780, and Samuel Rhoads resigned the next year. Thomas Wharton and Edward Pennington, although not members of the Board until well after the Hospital's founding, still put in seventeen years between them on that body, prior to their resignations in 1779. Although the majority of "new" Board members—those elected during the Revolutionary War—were Quakers, this new generation of Managers did not produce an Israel Pemberton or even a John Reynell. The Hospital would have to wait for the election of Samuel Coates to the Board in 1785, before the leadership void left by the death of the "King of the Quakers" could be filled. Nevertheless, a number of notable Managers began their services to the Hospital, during the Revolutionary War. Quaker Jonathan Shoemaker and non-Quakers Reynold Keene and Josiah Hewes all were elected to the Board of Managers in 1781. These three, as well as most of the other "new" Managers were, like their predecessors, primarily merchants.[19]

The Physicians

During the colonial period, the political views of the Quaker-dominated Board of Managers were often antithetical to the attitudes expressed by the Hospital's physicians. The contrasting views of both groups toward the College of Philadelphia, is a case in point. Perhaps the antithetical views of the physicians resulted from their religious attachments. Although some of the Hospital's physicians were Quakers prior to the Revolutionary War, Quakers were almost always a minority. In 1776, for example, none of the six physicians then serving the Hospital was a Friend. Thus when Quaker discipline demanded non-participation in revolutionary activities, the Hospital's physicians, in contrast to the Board, were not affected.

Sympathy for the rebel cause was the dominant feeling among the Hospital's physicians. Thomas Bond placed his services at the disposal of the revolutionaries, and aided his son, Thomas Bond, Jr., in "organizing the Medical Department of the Army." John Morgan was appointed "Director General and Chief Psysician" of the Continental Army Hospital in October of 1775, a position he held until January of 1777. Morgan was replaced by William Shippen, Jr., who would soon become a member of the staff of the Pennsylvania Hospital. Morgan's removal as "Director General" was, in no small part, the result of the vindictive activity of William Shippen, Jr. With the help of future Hospital physician, Benjamin Rush, Morgan struck back by bringing charges against Shippen, for malpractice and misconduct in office, and Shippen eventually resigned as "Director General" in 1781.[20] Although the Morgan-Shippen dispute did not directly affect the Hospital, the fact that both physicians were engaged in revolutionary activities, and then in personal polemics, limited the usefulness of both men to the Pennsylvania Hospital. Ostensibly, Morgan was on the Hospital staff throughout the Revolutionary War, with the exception of one year, but his attendance throughout much of the period was sporadic. William Shippen, Jr., was elected to the staff in the spring of 1778, but he never did attend Hospital patients during that year, and he was not re-elected until 1791. Even the elder Shippen was unable to fulfill his obligations to the Hospital because his "time was taken up in attending military hospitals."[21]

As in the case of the Board of Managers, the Revolutionary War witnessed the passing of the last of the Hospital's "old guard" physicians. Thomas Cadwalader, now sixty-seven years old, resigned in 1777; William Shippen, Sr., resigned the next year at sixty-six years of age. John Redman, who could number Benjamin Rush and John Morgan among his pupils, resigned from the Hospital in 1780 at the age of fifty-eight. The venerable founder of the Pennsylvania Hospital, Thomas Bond, did not resign until the spring of 1784, at the age of seventy-one, but the heavy work load of the Revolutionary years, must have done much to hasten retirement. John Morgan's reasons for stepping down were more a matter of principle than age. On April 28, 1783, the Board was told that two physicians of the Hospital—they were not named—were charging a fee of venereal patients from the House of Employment. The Board responded

> that in such instances, the physicians of this House are not entitled to, and therefore should not demand any fees or reward for their services.

Morgan, who was probably one of the two unnamed physicians collecting fees, immediately declined to serve the Hospital any longer. The Board thanked Morgan for his services and Morgan replied that he was always ready "upon any extraordinary emergencies to render" the Hospital "any further services in his power." Obviously, however, John Morgan had little use for the practice of treating venereal patients for free, because free care merely encouraged the very practice that spread the disease.[22]

The "new" physicians elected to replace the "old guard" offered medical degrees earned in America, as well as across the Atlantic. Both

James Hutchinson and Thomas Parke were elected to the Hospital's staff in 1777, after receiving their bachelor of medicine degrees from the Medical School of the College of Philadelphia. Both physicians, however, had crossed the Atlantic for further schooling, as had the other three "new" additions to the Hospital's medical staff. The influence of Edinburgh continued to be very significant, particularly after the election of Edinburgh-educated Benjamin Rush in 1783. John Jones, former student of Thomas Cadwalader and considered by some the foremost surgeon of his day, brought to the Hospital a M.D. degree from Rheims and experience at other European medical centers, when he was elected in 1780. The other "new" physician was William Shippen, Jr., who has already been spoken of in connection with anatomy courses at the Hospital, his role in the Medical School of the College of Philadelphia, and his position of "Director General" of the Continental Hospital. William Shippen, Jr., as previously pointed out, was elected to the Hospital staff in 1778, but did not actually serve that institution until after the American Revolution.[23]

The Apothecary

In April of 1776, James Dunlap resigned as apothecary. Previously, when in need of an apothecary, the Board would often write to John Fothergill in England for help. But now, because war existed between the mother country and the colonies, there was no possibility of recruiting a candidate from across the Atlantic. In March of the following year, John Story consented to assist in the apothecary shop—Story was already under Hospital employment as steward—at £25 additional salary per year. Story continued in his dual role of steward-apothecary until he was replaced in February of 1780 by Peter Yarnall. No reason is given for Story leaving the Hospital but, in the changing of apothecaries, the Hospital benefited financially. Story received £25 extra per year for his apothecary duties while Yarnall, initially at least, received only room and board. In November of 1780, John Bartram, Jr., applied for the apothecary position but Peter Yarnall decided to serve another year.

By August of 1782, Gustavus F. Kielman (spelled Kiellman in Sweden), student of Roland Martin at the University of Uppsala, and a Licentiate in Surgery at the Royal Seraphimer Hospital in Stockholm, Sweden, was hired as apothecary, at an undisclosed salary. In November, 1782, Kielman left for Cambridge, Massachusetts, where he taught botany and practiced medicine. He later returned to Sweden. The non-salaried James Hartley, who was recommended by Thomas Bond, replaced Kielman. Hartley remained as apothecary until the spring of 1784, when he was replaced at his own request.[24]

Because the "Elaboratory" had been rented to the Continental Army in 1778, the number of patients in the Hospital had decreased considerably, and with the flow of drugs from England interrupted by the war, one suspects that the position of apothecary was a good deal less demanding than in the pre-war years.

The Steward and Matron

In previous years the apothecary had often been the highest salaried employee of the Hospital, but during the war the steward usurped this honor. Continuing the exercise of executive power developed by George Weed, the Hospital's steward emerged from these trying times with his prerogatives still intact.

In the summer of 1775, steward John Saxton and his wife informed the Board that they would be leaving at the end of the year. John Story and his wife were hired to be the new steward and matron, respectively at the combined salary of £90 per year plus £10 additionally for their servant girl. The difficult times soon created morale problems for the Storys. Finally, in the spring of 1778, John Story "presented to the Board a paper containing sundry grievances . . ." that he supposed "himself to labour under. . . ." By the fall of the same year, the hard pressed board

"proposed . . . to take into consideration the propriety of discharging the present steward and matron on the expiration of their agreement."

This "consideration" may have been necessitated by financial imperatives rather than Board disapproval of the work of the Storys. By November of 1779, the Storys had left the Hospital's services and the Board now concerned itself with filling the vacant positions and settling John Story's account.[25]

By December, the Board had reduced the number of candidates for the steward's position to three, and on January 5, 1780, Joseph Henzey was hired. Whereas John Story filled the dual role of steward-apothecary, Joseph Henzey restricted himself to the single role of steward. Interestingly enough, the Board seemed little concerned with the office of matron, as it was rarely mentioned during the Revolutionary War. Evidently the matron's position was continuing its decline in significance, after once being the preeminent administrative position.

Perhaps conscious of his importance at the Hospital, Joseph Henzey asked for a raise at the end of his first year of employment, and the Board responded by increasing the Henzeys' combined salary from £50 to £70 in gold per year. When Joseph Henzey was subjected to militia fines, for not serving in the Revolution while on duty at the Hospital, the Board agreed ot pay the necessary taxes of £12 in specie and £6 in state money. At the end of his second year of service, Joseph Henzey informed the Board that he and his wife wanted another raise. The Board again saw fit to meet the request, and increased the Henzeys' salary to £90 per year. The same scenerio was repeated in January of 1783, with the Henzeys receiving another £20 salary increase.[26] Evidently the Board was well satisfied with their performance and would do anything in its power to retain them.

Other Members of the Staff

During the colonial period, the Hospital simultaneously employed two or three nurses. But with the subsequent decline of patients to approximately one-third or one-fourth their former number, only one nurse was needed. Probably a cleaning girl or maid, was also hired but no mention is made of her in the Hospital's records. Since the number of insane patients did not decline as dramatically as did non-insane patients, a cell keeper was still necessary. As in colonial times, the turnover in cell keepers was high. By 1781, the Managers were combining the cell keeping position with gardener.[27]

The Patients

As previously indicated, the number of patients decreased considerably during the Revolutionary period. Taking April as a specific date, the Hospital reported the following number of civilian patients in residence:

Year	Total Number of Resident Patients
1775	95
1776	62
1777	55
1778	28
1779	28
1780	41
1781	34
1782	26
1783	41

Even more alarming, was the decline in number of resident poor (non-paying) patients. Again a look at the figures for April point up a very revealing development:

Year	Total Number of Resident Patients	Number of Resident Poor Patients
1775	95	85
1776	62	60
1777	55	48
1778	28	22
1779	28	24
1780	41	33
1781	34	27
1782	26	15
1783	41	12

In short, the income from the Hospital's capital stock had so declined (see Appendix), that only a handful of poor patients could be supported, at the end of the Revolutionary period. Back in 1775, the revenue generated by the capital stock, supported seventy resident poor patients at a time (additional poor patients were financed by profits from pay patients and by borrowing from the capital stock). By April of 1783, the income from the capital stock had so declined that it had difficulty supporting twelve poor patients.[28]

Primarily an Insane Asylum

Perhaps just as alarming as the precipitous drop in poor patients, was the increase, percentage-wise, in insane patients. The following chart, from the month of April, clearly indicates that although the number of resident patients dramaticaly declined for the period 1775 to 1783, the number of resident insane patients declined only slightly.

Year	Number of Resident Patients	Number of Resident Insane Patients
1775	95	29
1776	62	19
1777	55	24
1778	28	20
1779	28	16
1780	41	20
1781	34	17
1782	26	18
1783	41	23

To summarize briefly, in April of 1775, insane patients represented about 31 percent of resident patients, but by April of 1783, that figure had risen to about 56 percent. The Pennsylvania Hospital, by the end of the American Revolution, had radically altered its nature. During the colonial period, careful restriction on the number of insane patients, allowed the Eighth and Pine institution to continue as a general hospital. But by the end of the American Revolution, the Pennsylvania Hospital was, primarily, an insane asylum. For the remainder of the eighteenth century, the majority of resident patients in the Pennsylvania Hospital, at any given time, would be classified as insane (see Appendix).[29]

The Hospital's weak financial situation explains the percentage increase in resident insane patients. While the overwhelming majority of physically ill patients were from poor families, who were unable to pay for their Hospital stay—slaves and indentured servants were an exception—the insane were often from families of some means, who could afford to pay. During the colonial period, for example, paying "lunatics" represented between 20 and 50 percent of the resident insane.[30] The continued reluctance of the Anglo-Saxon middle class, whether in London, Bristol or Philadelphia, to seek hospital admission for the treatment of physical illness, did not stop Philadelphia's "better sort" from paying, to send mentally ill relatives to Eighth and Pine, for safekeeping. The Hospital was a solution that was agreeable to everyone involved. Certain families in the Philadelphia area were rid of troublesome and emotionally disturbing relatives, while the Hospital collected badly needed revenue, to bolster its shaky financial foundation.

The decision to favor the admission of mentally ill, middle class patients was not formally recorded in the Managers' Minutes, but the figures on patients in residence, show clearly what was happening. In March of 1779, there were only three insane paying patients and thirteen insane poor (non-paying patients). By April of 1783, there were eighteen insane paying patients, and only eight insane poor patients. Not only had the Hospital opted for insane patients, but it had become quite discriminating, concerning the financial status of prospective insane patients. In short, the industrious poor, who had been well served by the Hospital in colonial times, found admission to the Hospital quite difficult during the later part of the Revolutionary period. The Board was sadly cognizant of this fact when, in 1780, it wrote John Fothergill

> that we have been under the sad necessity of refusing many proper objects of our charity.[31]

Out-Patients

During the colonial period, out-patients were greatly outnumbered by in-patients. During the Revolutionary period, out-patients outnumbered in-patients. In October of 1778, for example, there were some fifty out-patients treated, while in-patients for the same period, numbered less than forty. In May of the following year, forty-eight out-patients were treated and only slightly more than thirty in-patients. The fact that out-patients now outnumbered in-patients—indeed the total number of out-patients being treated seems to have increased since colonial times—can be ascribed to financial imperatives. The Hospital could continue to treat a large number of out-patients during the Revolutionary period because out-patients were not much of a financial drain on the Hospital. All that the Hospital paid for, in the treatment of such patients, was the medication prescribed by the Hospital's physicians.[32]

Deteriorating Conditions

Keeping pace with the decline in the number of resident patients, was the deteriorating treatment those patients received. By October of 1777, with Philadelphia under British occupation, and the Hospital housing many sick and wounded British soldiers, the Hospital's Board was informed by the sitting Managers that all was not well. The latter noted laconically that the patients are as well taken care of as the circumstances of the times will admit of.

Evidently, the insane suffered greatly because the basement section of the Hospital, where many of them were housed, was not heated. By the spring of 1778, steward John Story complained to the Board, that many of the patients were in want of clothing. In August of 1778, the sitting Managers made known an urgent need for new "beds and bedding," but no relief was found, and the same appeal was repeated two months later. By January 25, 1779, the situation seems to have improved, as the Board was told that "the patients are more comfortably provided for than some time past." The insane, however, were suffering from cold, because of broken windows in their cells. Although Continental soldiers were accommodated in some of the Hospital's beds during the spring of 1779, conditions for most civilian patients remained relatively tolerable, and throughout the late spring and summer of 1779, the rooms of the Hospital were described as "pretty clean."

In the summer of 1780, Dr. Morgan reported a shortage of drugs, and the following winter, the Hospital was again in need of bedding, and a cell keeper. All of these problems were solved within a few months. A committee of the Board raised £40 to replenish the drug supply, a cell keeper was employed, and eight beds and thirty-one blankets were purchased. In October of 1781, the sitting Managers reported that the House was now "clean and in good order."[33] For the remainder of the Revolutionary period, conditions in the Hospital would be summarized as "clean and in good order." "Clean and in good order" indicates improved conditions for the Hospital's patients by 1782 and 1783, and mortality statistics support this conclusion.

During the colonial period, mortality among patients admitted to the Hospital was about 12 percent. For the three years prior to the Revolution (1773–1775), the mortality rate rose to 13 percent. For the revolutionary period the mortality rate climbed to slightly less than 18 percent, reflecting the deteriorating conditions in the Hospital during those years (1776–1783). But by 1782, the mortality rate supported the sitting Managers' optimistic reports about improving conditions, with a 3 percent decrease from the previous year. The combined mortality rate for the final two years of the Revolutionary period (1782 and 1783), actually dropped to about 12 percent, which matched the overall rate for the colonial period.[34] If the preservation of the life of its patients is a hospital's measuring rod, the Pennsylvania Hospital was functioning as effectively at the end of the American Revolution, as it had, prior to that struggle. In the number, type of affliction and class background of its patients, however, the Hospital had not returned to its pre-war pattern.

Chapter 5

Managing During the
Recovery Years, 1784-1801

THE END OF the American Revolution brought increased participation in humanitarian reforms by Philadelphia Quakers. Prison reform, in particular, drew attention from individual Quakers, causing the formation of the Philadelphia Society for Alleviating the Miseries of Public Prisons (later the Pennsylvania Prison Society). Philadelphia Quakers, along with their brethren elsewhere, were also in the forefront of abolitionist societies and other groups to improve the lot of the Negro.[1] It was in keeping with this humanitarian surge, that a new generation of Quakers, which had reached maturity during the war years, turned its energies to aiding the recovery of the Pennsylvania Hospital, from the debilitating effects of the Revolutionary War. In the effort to resurrect the stricken Hospital, however, the Quaker community found itself increasingly dependent on Philadelphia's non-Quaker population.

By the end of the Revolution, strained relations between the Quaker community and other Pennsylvanians had somewhat abated. Most of the Friendly community now accepted the new revolutionary government and took their places as loyal citizens in the young republic. With Philadelphians and other Pennsylvanians no longer suspicious of Quaker intentions, one might suppose that new contributions to the Pennsylvania Hospital—held back during the war years because of antipathy towards Quakers, and thus towards institutions dominated by Quakers—would reach prewar levels. An optimistic observer might have predicted that, within a few years, the Hospital would be supporting as many resident poor patients as in its golden years, just prior to the Revolution. Unfortunately, there was another spirit abroad that delayed and retarded the recovery of the Hospital, and it wouldn't be until well into the nineteenth century, that the Hospital supported the number of resident poor patients cared for in 1775.

This "new" spirit, or attitude, which had such a negative effect on the Hospital, seemed to permeate the entire nation after the Revolution; and because of it, useful and humanitarian organizations and institutions of all types, did not flourish. Moreau de St. Méry pointed this out in his visit to Philadelphia in the mid-1790's, and further noted that

"any attempt to arouse interest in public welfare has too often been impeded by the sluggishness and the heedlessness natural to Americans."

Perhaps St. Méry's explanation for American lack of progress in this area is too simplistic to be wholly satisfying, but his general observation on the lack of flourishing philanthropic institutions, seems to be fairly accurate. Across the new republic, a number of colleges were founded during the two postwar decades, only to founder, for a number of years. The Philadelphia Almshouse and the University of Pennsylvania, which, along with the Hospital, were Philadelphia's leading philanthropic institutions, also found it difficult going during this period. Evidently, most Americans were now less willing to support, or less capable of supporting, institutional philanthropy, than in late colonial times.[2]

The Board of Managers

In the post-Revolutionary period, Quaker hegemony over the Hospital was less certain than in previous years. For the first time since the founding of the Hospital, the percentage of Managers who were Friends, fell below 50 percent. From 1784 to 1801 some thirty-four different men served as Managers, and only sixteen, or 47 percent, were Quakers. This compared with figures of 57 percent, for the colonial period, and 67 percent, for the Revolutionary period. If one counts only the Managers who served five years or better—again these would probably be the most influential Managers—the Quaker figure for 1784 to 1801 climbs to 59 percent, but that is still far short of the 80 percent figure, for the colonial period, or the 73 percent figure, for the Revolutionary years.[3]

Even more than in colonial times the Managers in the post-Revolutionary period tended to be merchants, although they were not as prominent members of the mercantile community, as were their predecessors.[4] Stephen Noyes Winslow, in his *Biographies of Success Philadelphia Merchants* (post-Revolutionary merchants), finds only three of the thirty-four Managers who served during the recovery period, worthy of treatment. One suspects that a comparable study of Philadelphia's colonial mercantile community, would include a considerably larger number of Managers. Henry Simpson's *Lives of Eminent Philadelphians Now Deceased* (1859), lists twelve Managers, who served the Hospital during its first half century. Eight served the Hospital prior to the Revolution, while only four were Managers after that time. In short, the Hospital was no longer drawing its Managers, primarily, from the ranks of Philadelphia's wealthiest, and most distinguished citizens. Rather, it was now turning to a level of society that was wealthy but not really aristocratic, to a group that exercised some influence, but did not represent the political leadership of the city, or the state. No longer did the Hospital have at its disposal the advice of the likes of Thomas Bond, Benjamin Franklin, Israel Pemberton, John Reynell and William Logan. It was obvious that Philadelphia's elite was occupied with other, more pressing problems during the post-Revolutionary period.

Although the Hospital no longer could count a large number of legislators or merchant princes on its Board, this did not mean that the dedication and zeal of the Managers was any less than before independence. The fact that Board membership was less and less drawn from Philadelphia's elite, may have been advantageous, because recovery from the hardships imposed by war, demanded more than dilettantism from the Managers. The Hospital needed men who would not be distracted by interests, other than the welfare of the patients at Eighth and Pine.

Samuel Coates

Back in 1765, Israel Pemberton gave up most of his outside activities in order to concentrate on Hospital affairs, as well as on some other humanitarian interests. In 1785, Samuel Coates, a thirty-six year old Quaker merchant, was elected to the Board. Within a few years this new Manager would duplicate Pemberton's willingness to abandon most of his other interests for the sake of the Hospital, and would fill the leadership role once exercised by the "King of the Quakers."

Samuel Coates lost both parents at an early age and was taken in by his uncle, John Reynell, who was president of the Hospital's Board from 1757 to 1781. After a good classical and business education, young Coates entered into mercantile activities, under his uncle's wing. Obviously idolizing his uncle—Coates would name his first born, John Reynell Coates, and his last born, Reynell Coates—it was only natural that young Samuel would wish to emulate his uncle's commitment to the Hospital.

Initially successful as a merchant, Coates turned increasingly to civic commitments that included, in addition to the Pennsylvania Hospital, the Philadelphia Quaker schools, the Library Company of Philadelphia and, as a director, the First Bank of the United States. A portrait by Thomas Sully in 1813 presents the then sixty-five year old Manager.

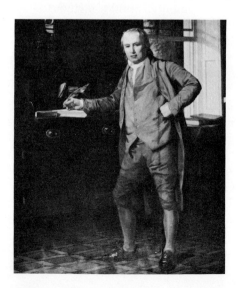

Although very interested in the Hospital from the beginning, Coates continued to show almost equal interest in his mercantile pursuits until the onslaught of the yellow fever epidemic in 1793. From that year, until cataracts on both eyes forced retirement, Coates devoted the major part of his energy to philanthropic interests, with the Hospital taking up most of his time. A year after his election to the Board, Coates was chosen secretary, and served in that position until 1812, when he was elected president of the Board. He held the latter position until his failing eyesight forced him to step down in 1825. For forty-one years this indefatigable Quaker served the Hospital, and upon his death in 1830, the Board of Managers, in a memorial, stated that

> "no individual ever connected with the administration of the Hospital bestowed as much personal attention upon its affairs. . . ."

In fact, Coates bestowed so much personal attention on the Hospital that his business ventures ceased, and his once wealthy estate so declined by the time of his death, that only a "small residue" was left for his family.[5]

Like Israel Pemberton before him, Samuel Coates dominated Hospital proceedings by force of personality and willingness to work. Within a short interval after election to the Board in 1785, his influence was obvious, as his name appeared on all of the important committees, and significant meetings took place in his home. Respect for Coates by his fellow Managers can be seen in Coates' election, in 1786, to the position of secretary—this was the position initially held by Franklin, during the Hospital's first year—and in the willingness of the Board to adjourn a meeting in October of 1787, because Lydia Coates, Samuel's first wife, had died two days earlier.

Coates was particularly interested in the insane. He kept a memorandum book in which he recorded his observations on particular insane cases. Perhaps this interest in the insane was kindled by Coates' friendship with Benjamin Rush, who also took a special interest in mental illness. But more likely, this interest went back to an incident in early childhood. A maid-servant, who previously had shown some signs of "derangement," seized the six week old Samuel from his Philadelphia home and stole away, unobserved. The kidnapped infant was eventually rescued, but only after an attempt by the deranged kidnapper, to hurl young Samuel from a second story window, was narrowly averted. No doubt this curious and frightening incident created in Samuel Coates, a certain curiosity about mental illness.[6]

There were other Managers whose services were important to the Hospital from 1784 to 1801. Although born in New Jersey, merchant Josiah Hewes moved to Philadelphia, and was elected Manager in 1781, and President in 1790. Hewes continued as President until Samuel Coates replaced him in 1812. Probably the best memorial to Josiah Hewes was the completion of the center and west wing of the Hospital during his presidency. Others who, because of activities on various committees, and years of service on the Board, deserve mention, include sea captain-merchant Nathaniel Falconer and merchant and Quaker convert Elliston Perot.[7]

Financial Recovery

In 1779 a despairing John Pemberton wrote James Fothergill of the "very languishing state" of the Hospital, and of his own fear that the Hospital "can not long be supported." But somehow the Hospital survived, and even improved its financial status, and the conditions under which its patients lived. Thus, when Dr. Johann David Schoepf visited the Hospital in 1783, he found one ward

> high, airy and long and well . . . kept, like the whole establishment in a very cleanly state.

However, Schoepf also found that, because of continued financial weakness—albeit not as serious as four years earlier—the Hospital could not care for "the established number of sick."[8]

In 1784, the productive capital stock of the Hospital was just barely over £10,000, producing an income from rents and interest, of £722. That same year, other sources of income such as contributions, legacies, charity boxes, board of paying patients, etc., amounted to approximately £1,287, giving the Hospital a total income for 1784 of £2,009. Operating expenses for the same period, amounted to £110 more than income. What the Managers had to do immediately was to balance income with operating expenses.[9] This could be accomplished by simultaneously cutting back on expenses and increasing the income-producing capital stock.

Using a previously successful method of fund raising, the Board made ready to publish abstracts of accounts of the Hospital, for the years 1775 and 1783, in order to contrast the financial position of the Hospital, before and after the American Revolution. Initially, this Board seemed to lack the energy of previous Boards and moved very slowly to meet the Hospital's financial problems; but with the election of Samuel Coates, in July of the following year, the Board began to move with new vigor. In October, it decided to go to the public for further donations, and a committee was appointed to publish an introductory piece in the newspapers. Then, on March 2, 1786, the Board assigned a committee to find out

> "the causes from whence the great expenses of the house arises, and also to recommend some general plan for the government thereof, and to inspect the accounts now laid before the board by the steward."

Twenty-eight days later, the Committee on Economy, made up of Andrew Doz, Reynold Keene and Samuel Coates, presented their report to the Board. To save money, the committee recommended that the salaries of the steward and matron be cut back, the amount of liquor served to patients be greatly reduced, baking be done on the premises, as well as soap making, and that the

"Managers carefully . . . check the steward's market expenses as we find now and then articles we think too luxurious and expensive for the Hospital to admit."

As a result of the above recommendations, the combined salary of the matron and steward was reduced from £110 per year to £80 per year, liquor was restricted to use only if prescribed by one of the physicians, and candles and soap were produced on the grounds.[10]

After having done what it could to reduce costs, the Board continued its drive to solicit increased contributions from the public. Publicity, in the form of newspaper articles, continued to be the method used to encourage contributions. Results were not spectacular, but by 1796, productive capital stock was up to £18,305 which generated an income that year of £1,313. But not all of the increase in capital stock could be credited to individual contributions.[11]

Back in 1773, the Hospital had been able to realize £11,990 (£8,637 sterling) from the unclaimed shares of the Pennsylvania Land Company. The Revolution intervened, preventing the Hospital from realizing even more from this windfall. With the end of hostilities, the Managers turned again to such British friends as David Barclay, for aid in collecting money belonging to the Hospital, but still in the hands of the trustees of the defunct Pennsylvania Land Company. Finally, in 1787, an additional £917.19.5 was received from this source.[12]

Benefit performances, such as the six lectures by educator, lexicographer and editor Noah Webster, and a concert of sacred music at a German Reformed church, added to the Hospital's coffers. Money signers continued the practice begun in colonial times, of turning their gains over to the Hospital and, in 1787, the Hospital received £188 from signers.[13]

To protect and enlarge revenues from the growing capital stock, the Managers made certain that the payment of cheap currency in return for dear money, which had caused the near financial collapse of the Hospital during the Revolution, would not be repeated. Even state currency, which had not undergone the cataclysmic depreciation experienced by Continental notes during the Revolution, was not to be trusted. Income producing loans were made with state paper, but were to be repaid in specie. Even this cautious approach was not enough to satisfy the uneasy Board, and in June of 1785, the Hospital's treasurer was directed to sell the state money belonging to the Hospital "on the best terms he can."[14]

To produce as much income as possible from the growing capital stock was paramount. Prior to the Revolution, the Managers had loaned out, at interest, most of the Hospital's liquid capital. During the postwar period, however, the Managers began to invest rather heavily in ground rentals. The Hospital would purchase from the owner of a particular piece of property, the right to collect the ground rent for a period of years—usually sixteen—after which time the ground rents would revert back to the property owner. Generally this arrangement helped property owners in immediate need of sizeable amounts of cash, and worked out to the Hospital's benefit, because the total rents collected exceeded the initial outlay to the property owner.

By 1795, the Hospital was investing slightly more of its liquid capital in ground rentals than in loans, and for good reason. Usually, the ground rentals returned about 6 percent annually on the capital invested, whereas loans produced only about a 5 percent annual return. Another rather interesting innovation saw the Managers investing—small sums to be sure—in the Insurance Company of North America and the Philadelphia Water Works. From these rather meager investments (they totaled no more than £412 by 1801) a tradition of investing in corporations was begun.[15]

It was one thing to loan out money, or invest in ground rentals, and quite a different matter to collect the payments due. The Board spent long hours in dealing with the problem of delinquent rents and overdue repayments of loans. Litigation was often the only alternative open to the Hospital when appeals to charitable, noble and honest sentiments failed. By August of 1786

"the loss of the Institution sustained by diverse persons who are indebted for interest, rent, etc., and who neglect to pay the same in due time . . ."

caused the Board to appoint a committee of Reynold Keene, Joseph Paschall and Samuel Coates "to sue all such delinquents." Even another charitable institution did not escape the energetic prosecution of Keene, Paschall and Coates. The Philadelphia Almshouse (Bettering House or House of Employment) owed the Hospital some £905 by 1789—the particulars of this case will be taken up later in this chapter—and, after bringing legal action against the same, the initial debt, plus subsequent debts were paid to the Hospital in 1791.[16] As vigorous as were the activities of the Board in soliciting contributions and collecting debts, annual operating expenses continued to climb more rapidly than the income generated by the capital stock (see Appendix).

From the very beginning of the Hospital, a dynamic tension existed between the impulse to restrict patients to deserving sick-poor who were judged "curable," and the example set by the Good Samaritan, of helping all those in need, regardless of the character of the victim, or the nature of his disease. Indeed, within a few years of its founding, the Hospital chose the Good Samaritan for its official seal. Therefore, despite the fact that it did cater to the "curable industrious poor," the Hospital did not totally ignore the victims of incurable afflictions. The practice of admitting some "incurable" insane patients, dating back to the first years of the Hospital, was continued into the nineteenth century, but not without public criticism. After all, it made more sense to spend limited funds on the curable, because they, once healed, could again make constructive contributions to society.

In a newspaper article written for public consumption in 1785, the Managers aired this conundrum, and then justified retaining some incurable patients, "most of whom are lunaticks," because these incurables "have neither friends to visit them or means to clothe them with necessary clothing." The article did admit, however, that the incurable "are a continuous burthen, . . ." and, if only such patients could find shelter somewhere else, the purpose of the Hospital (healing the sick) could be carried out at less expense.[17] Some fifteen years later, the case of William Ray underlined the basic humanitarian concern that characterized the Board. Ray, suffering from an abdomen wound, was admitted even though his case was incurable. Doctor Barton, the attending physician who admitted Ray, was sternly scolded by the Board. After pointing out that, under the rules of admission the only incurables admitted were lunatics, the Board allowed, however, that

> "to carry this rule in the present case into a strict execution might occasion the immediate death of William Ray, for which reason the Managers consent, though reluctantly, to let him remain in the House."

Evidently the Hospital's employees were also beneficiaries of the Board's humanitarian bent. Steward Joseph Henzey was "struck with the palsy" in 1796 and rendered incapable of further serving the Hospital. The Board allowed the stricken steward to continue to collect his salary, until a new steward could be hired. The Board also allowed Henzey to remain in the Hospital, free of charge for a limited time and, thereafter, at a charge of five shillings per week, which was considerably less than other paying patients were charged.[18]

In the face of rising costs, the Board's attempt to hold down expenses was unsuccessful. In 1784, for example, the combined outlay for the apothecary shop and for Hospital employees' wages, amounted to about £314. Nine years later, with about the same number of patients in the Hospital, combined costs of the two above cited items, soared to almost £740. During that same span, household expenses (primarily food and fuel) increased by one third. The rising costs of goods and services, meant an increase in cost per patient, to the Hospital. During the last decade of the colonial period, the cost of boarding and caring for each patient, averaged out to about seven shillings per week. By 1793, the cost per patient had increased to twelve shillings, six pence per week.

This 83 percent increase in cost per patient put a tremendous burden on the Hospital's capital stock. Less than £400 of capital stock could support one poor patient, for an entire year in 1775. In 1793, almost £700 was needed to do the same job (this is based on the assumption that invested capital stock produced somewhere between a 5 and 6 percent return). In order for the capital stock of the 1790's to match the "real" productiveness of the capital stock of the colonial period, the former had to exceed the latter by some 80 to 90 percent. In short, to support the Hospital in the style to which it was accustomed during its early years, the capital stock had to reach the £36,000-£38,000 range in the 1790's.[19] It never came close (see Appendix).

Additions and Repairs

Constant repairs and additions to the physical property consumed a great deal of the Board's attention. Intent on protecting the block that the Hospital occupied, the Managers continued the policy, begun during the colonial era, of buying up surrounding tracts of land. Prior to the Revolution, the greater part of the square, directly west of the Hospital, was divided between the Hospital and the Almshouse. During that same period, the Hospital acquired most of the square directly to the east. By 1788, Hospital ownership of the entire block to the east, was completed and the Board turned its attention to acquiring, piecemeal, the block to the south. But purchase of this block did not begin until 1801, and was not completed until 1831.

Because maintenance work had been neglected during the war years, structural repairs were urgent. In 1786, the Board after "considering the ruinous condition of the building will soon be in without painting," unanimously agreed that a paint job was necessary, and Samuel Coates was assigned to purchase the oil. By April of the following year the building, inside and out, was under a new coat of paint. Other repairs and additions completed about the same time, included a new shed over the cells for the insane, and a gutter and stone pavement in front of the Hospital wall, on Eighth Street. In 1789, a smokehouse was thought necessary and the sitting Managers were instructed to get one built "in such a part of the lot as they apprehend is most convenient." Another shed was added in 1791, and an icehouse in 1794.[20]

The Center Building and West Wing

All of the above real estate and construction decisions were dwarfed by the most important construction decision of the period: the resolve to complete the original design for the Hospital, by erecting a west wing, and a center building. Although the total number of patients housed in the Hospital had decreased since colonial times, the number of insane patients had not, and indeed, would have probably increased, if there were cells enough to house them (see Appendix).

Fifteen cells in the basement floor, housed the most serious cases of insanity, while the remainder of the insane had to be housed with the other patients, in the two wards, and private rooms above. Placing some of the insane in the wards was undesirable, but no other alternative seemed possible, particularly, in view of the constant increase of "lunatics," among the populace of the state, due to the "increase of inhabitants . . . as well as by many other causes." Thus, in 1792, the Managers and Physicians decided that

an extension of the House, as nearly as possible to agree with the original plan, admitting only of such alternatives as will more conveniently accommodate the lunatics is indispensably needful . . .

The obvious source of funds for such a venture was the state legislature, and a committee of the Board, which included the indefatigable Samuel Coates, made ready a petition to the legislature, requesting assistance to enable the Contributors

"to . . . [build] in such manner, as to answer the humane intentions of its [the Hospital's] original founders." [21]

Because the state judiciary was often involved in deciding the fate of lunatics, the Board's committee approached three judges of the State Supreme Court for support. Judges Thomas McKean, William Bradford and Edward Shippen (cousin to Hospital physician William Shippen, Jr.,) offered to introduce the committee's petition to the Assembly, provided that

"if the money was granted, and the building extended, in consequence of our joint applications, a clause should be inserted to provide, that they the judges, should have free liberty, to commit the lunatics, therein, from every part of the state, without the let or hindrance of any of the Managers."

But this request reminded the Managers of the Proprietor—Managers' dispute of the 1750's, because the judges were attempting to usurp the prerogatives of the Board, in much the same fashion unsuccessfully pursued by Thomas Penn, during the Hospital's first decade. The analogy between Thomas Penn and the three judges cannot be carried too far, however, because the latter group did promise, if their proposal was rejected,

"to cooperate . . . in applying for the grant as private gentlemen, but not as judges of the Supreme Court."

The Board unanimously rejected the proposal of the three judges but did hold them to their promise, to exert themselves as "private gentlemen", on behalf of the Hospital.

The Managers then presented a petition to the legislature and the legislature appointed a committee to visit the Hospital. The committee gave good grades to the Hospital on almost all counts, but did find housing for lunatics unsatisfactory because there were not enough cells to hold them all. Acting upon the committee's recommendation, the legislature granted £10,000 ($26,666.67) to the Hospital, out of arrears due the Commonwealth under the Loan Office Act of February 26, 1773. Periodic payments were made to the Hospital by the Loan Office until 1804, when the above mentioned sum had been reached. By the same act that gave the Hospital £10,000 of the money due the Loan Office, the Assembly provided that all unclaimed dividends of "Bankrupt's Estates" were to be paid to the Hospital. Approximately $27,000 was realized from this source, through two payments from the Commissioners in Bankruptcy to the Hospital in 1795 and 1796.[22]

Buoyed by the government grants of 1793, the Managers turned to planning the new additions. The original plan by Samuel Rhoads was to be followed as nearly as possible, although architectural trends seemed to point to some adjustments. Master builder David Evans, member of the Carpenters' Company and, in 1788–1789, a participant in the construction of Library Hall on Fifth Street—the Library of the American Philosophical Society occupies the site of Library Hall and is an architectural facsimile—was asked to give an estimate of the costs of the new additions. In January of 1794, Evans submitted in writing the opinion that

> "the additional buildings, may all be finished in the outside, and the walls of the area be built, and all the floors laid, for ten thousand pounds [approximately $26,667.00], exclusive of the stone steps and curbstones round the area, and the frontispiece to the outside door."

Evans also sent along "a ground plan for the whole," drawn by his son David Evans, Jr., which included an added estimate of £3,309, for the internal completion of the western wing.[23]

The Managers, as they were required to do in such weighty matters, brought the proposal for the additional buildings before the Contributors and received a green light. At the Contributor's meeting, it was also resolved

> "that the western wing extend in width six feet more than the present ward [eastern wing]"

—in the actual construction, another foot was added—so as to admit two rows of cells to a floor. The west wing needed the large number of cells that this arrangement would provide, because that wing was to house, exclusively, the insane. The Contributor's meeting also decided that

> "the House be finished with a dome, and the south front thereof, with six marble pilasters, agreeable to the elevation now exhibited."

A building committee composed of Managers Thomas Morris, Samuel Clark, Thomas Penrose, Bartholomew Wistar and Joseph Paschall, was formed at the next Board meeting and charged with procuring building materials and digging the foundations, as early as possible, in the spring of 1794, "and to continue building so as to enclose the whole, in the ensuing fall." Unfortunately there were no master builders on the Board at this time—Samuel Rhoads and Joseph Fox had long since died—and so the Board

> "agreed that one carpenter shall be engaged as a principal [supervisor] to undertake the whole buildings with liberty to employ his own workmen. . . ."

The "principal" was to be responsible only to the Board.

The building committee nominated, and the Board voted unanimously, in favor of David Evans, Jr., for the position of "principal" carpenter, and asked him to draw up the terms under which he would "undertake the work." Evans agreed to do the "whole of the carpenter's work, at the old printed book of prices," and if the carpenter's book prices increased by 25 percent, as he expected they would in the near future, his charge would not increase more than 10 percent. David Evans, Sr., was very pleased that the Board decided on his son, and because of his concern for the interests of his son, and the welfare of the Hospital, offered "to superintend the work without any compensation." The Board accepted the senior Evans' offer.[24]

By late February of 1794, the building committee realized its plans for putting up the entire outside structures of the two new buildings, and enclosing them before the onslaught of the next winter, were too ambitious. Now, in a more practical frame of mind, the building committee proposed that only the cellar be dug, and walled up "in the ensuing season. . . ." The Board approved the new proposal and work began in the spring of 1794. In need of stone for a basement in the center house, the alert Managers noted that the state government was taking down part of the fort at Mud Island. In June of 1794, the Managers sent a request to Governor Thomas Mifflin, asking for "a preference in the sale of the resulting stone." The Hospital was eventually able to procure some of the stone from Mud Island, but not a sufficient amount "to carry up the basement stories of the center house, . . ." and the building committee was forced to buy additional stone, at market price.[25]

By the spring of 1795 the foundations of the two new buildings had been laid, but prices for labor and materials were climbing. A committee from the Assembly, after visiting the Hospital, noted

> "the unexampled rise in the price of labour and materials which has taken place,"

and the fact that the action taken by the legislature in April 11, 1793 (loan office payments and bankruptcy dividends already spoken of), was not as helpful as might first appear, because only a total of £7,127 had been realized to date. By late November, 1795, rising costs made it obvious that the legislative grant of 1793 was insufficient for the completion of the new buildings, and the Board sent a letter to Governor Mifflin, requesting that the Governor "in general terms . . . represent to the next assembly . . ." the need for further financial aid

> "as may be sufficient to complete the buildings; without which the work that is already done will be of no advantage."

At the time of the Board's new request for government aid, total construction costs had almost reached the £12,000 level.

So far, the western wing had been "covered" and some progress had been made in "carrying up the center house," but at the cost of exhausting all of the money received from the Loan Office Act (some £7,696

had been received by early December, 1795), and of borrowing some
£1,863 from the capital stock. If aid were not forthcoming from the
legislature, the Board had the choice of abandoning the partly constructed
new buildings, or finishing them at the cost of seriously depleting the
capital stock. Faced with these two untenable options, the Board sent a
memorial to the legislature asking for an additional grant of £15,000
"to finish the buildings."[26]

On April 2, 1796, the Managers were informed that a bill granting
$25,000 to the Hospital had passed both Houses of the legislature, and
was signed by the Governor. Although somewhat less than they asked
for—$25,000 equaled a little less than £10,000—no initial public com-
plaints seem to have been made by the Managers. By May, however, the
Managers noted that the

> "the prices of materials continuing to increase beyond all our calculations and
> the late grant of the assembly being inadequate to extend the buildings on
> the plan that has been contemplated by the Contributors, it is agreed to
> suspend the buildings of the Center House, except to open a communication
> with the Western Division until further order is taken therein."

The Board even considered calling a meeting of the Contributors, to
determine whether or not the "marble fronts" and pilasters should be
disposed with. By January 30, 1797, the possibility of finishing the center
building looked even bleaker, as the Board estimated that outside help
of at least £5,675 was necessary for completion, and that was only if no
increase in construction costs took place.

A few months earlier, Governor Mifflin visited the Hospital and signi-
fied his willingness to recommend to the legislature, that a further sum
be granted to the Hospital, in order to complete the center building. But,
unknown to the Board, the state legislature, in April of 1796, had made
its last grant to the brick institution on Eighth and Pine. Despite repeated
memorials to the Governor and the legislature, in future years the Hospital would have to look, almost exclusively, to private philanthropy for
support.[27]

To add to the Board's anxiety, in early 1797, David Evans, Jr., demanded "an addition of thirty-two pounds in the hundred on the old book
prices . . ." for the wages due the carpenters under his supervision. The
Board pointed out that such a radical increase was contrary to the promise, made three years earlier, by Evans that his charge would never exceed
10 percent of the "old book prices." The Board went on to point out that
10 percent of the old prices was the "utmost" that he could claim, and
the dispute went to an impartial board for settlement. Just how the issue
was settled, and who made up the "impartial board", is not clear. We do
know that David Evans, Jr., continued on the job, and even boarded at
the Hospital, during the yellow fever epidemic of 1797. Evans "took the
yellow fever the day after he came into the House" and, after being
moved to the "westernmost apartments of the new building," was cured.

By December 28, 1797, the western wing was finished and outfitted with wards "in a stile of superior consequence for the accommodation of lunatic patients." By the same date, the center building

"designed for the residence of the officers and servants of the Family and for other necessary purposes,"

had been "raised and partly enclosed." Whether or not to proceed with the construction of a dome over the center building, was the next issue confronting the Hospital, and a special meeting of the Contributors was convened on July 9, 1798. The Contributors were informed that, in 1794 they had decided to finish the center house with a dome, but that the building commitee found it "difficult to adopt any dome to the present style of the front." Furthermore, the building committee assured the Contributors that the operating room, planned for the third floor, would receive just "as good a light from the platform of the roof. . . ." The Contributors followed the suggestion of the building committee and

"resolved, that the dome be omitted and the skylight finished with a light railing."

A temporary halt from lack of funds put off finishing the rooms in the center building for a couple of years, and it was not until 1804 that all of the rooms in the center building were completed as planned.[28]

The two new structures, (the center building and west wing) joined with the original Hospital building (east wing), to form a symetrically balanced structure, along the lines envisioned by Samuel Rhoads' original plan of 1755. The west wing almost duplicated the east wing, except that the west wing was some seven feet wider and was topped by a slightly different cupola. The center building, on the other hand, featured a facade and a skylight not envisioned by Rhoads. Rhoads' original design called for a facade that featured the use of decorative coins, belt courses delineating each floor, and a projecting core topped by a triangular pediment, which broke the flat surface of the front of the center building. Despite the above mentioned embellishments, Rhoads' design projected a utilitarian, almost austere, visage.

By contrast, the newly completed center building presented a less austere facade. The first floor was fronted with stone, while the second and third had their reddish-brown brick faces interrupted, at regular intervals, by Corinthian pilasters topped by a triangular pediment, a prominent balustrade, and a circular skylight, with its own balustrade, visible from the ground. Four recessed, gracefully rounded at-the-top windows, broke the first floor's stone facade and set off an attractive entrance. Marble steps, bracketed by two iron grillwork railings, led up to a recessed door, topped by a rising sun transom. Whereas Rhoads' design could be best characterized as early Georgian, the new center building's facade revealed the more sophisticated style of the Federal period. (See the next page for the Hospital as an engraving presented it in 1802.)[29]

In contrast with the east and west wings, the center building at least in its facade, may have been inspired by a specific contemporary structure. In 1790, work was completed on Library Hall, but not before one of the carpenters fell from a three-story scaffold and was seriously injured. The unlucky craftsman was David Evans, Sr., and the structure he was working on bore, in its facade, a striking resemblance to the second and third floors of the Hospital's center building. Although David Evans, Sr.,

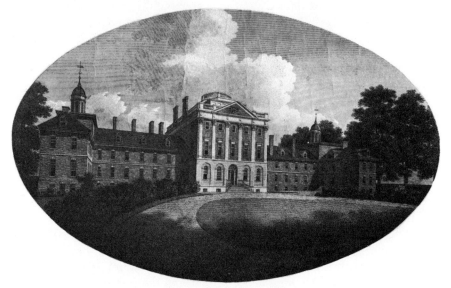

The Hospital in 1802.

was not the architect of Library Hall—William Thornton, physician turned architect, designed that structure—he was, obviously, very familiar with its facade, as was his son, David Evans, Jr., who drew up the initial plans for the Hospital's west wing and center building. Moreover, the Board of Directors of the Library Company included, in 1789, Hospital Managers Joseph Paschall and Josiah Hewes, while Library Company director Thomas Morris would be elected Hospital Manager, in 1795. Even Thomas Parke, Hospital physician, was a Library director, while Hospital Manager and secretary, Samuel Coates, was also secretary of the Library Company. Thus the new Library Company building,

> "displaying elements of the Adamesque-Federal style then coming into vogue in Philadelphia,"

was extremely familiar to the Hospital community and was probably the Philadelphia prototype for the center building's facade.[30]

The interior of the new west wing differed from the east wing in being some seven feet wider, and in being divided into individual rooms, off of a long hallway. The latter arrangement was, of course, dictated by the decision to use the west wing exclusively for the insane. The cupola which topped the west wing seemed, to the casual observer, to be just another decorative embellishment. To the residents of the Hospital, however, this cupola, as well as its counterpart atop the east wing, afforded "a secure way out in case of fire." All of the insane were moved out of the basement cells in the east wing, and that structure, by 1797, housed only the physically ill, in its two open wards on the first and second floors. The center building acted as a buffer, by shielding the physically ill from the disturbing cries of the insane. The first floor of the center building became the administrative center, and provided room for the apothecary shop, and living quarters for some of the Hospital staff, as well as the home for the Hospital Library, from 1800 to 1807. The operating room amphitheatre, which would not be completed, and ready for use until 1804, was on the third floor.

By the end of 1801, the Hospital was structurally sound, even though some inside work on the center building remained to be completed. Where, one immediately asks, did the money come from to pay for all of the new construction? By December of 1801, construction costs had reached $84,000, only $66,000 of which had been given by the legislature. Again the Managers, as they had throughout much of the Hospital's history, exhibited a great deal of resourcefulness. By borrowing heavily, they were able to satisfy the Hospital's creditors—by January of 1801 the Managers had already borrowed some $17,000—and, at the same time, insured the completion of the new buildings.[31] Presenting Philadelphians with a "fait accompli" seemed to make good "money raising" sense, because few Philadelphians, who ventured forth for a country outing via Pine Street, could deny that certain philanthropic sentiments were conjured up by the splendid sight of the newly completed Hospital.

Relations With the Almshouse

Many resident Hospital patients were not unused to institutional care. Some had previously resided in the Philadelphia Almshouse, which was located only one block west of the Hospital. Relations between these two institutions occupied a great deal of the Board's time and, therefore, deserve some treatment.

In 1731 or 1732, the Philadelphia Almshouse was erected on Third and Spruce Streets, after the colonial legislature loaned the city £1,000

> to be applied to the purchase of ground and erection of an Almshouse for the use of the poor of the city.

Because some of the poor who were housed there were sick or insane, John W. Croskey, historian of the Philadelphia General Hospital, which traces its roots back to the Almshouse, maintains that the building on Third and Spruce functioned as the first hospital in America. D. Hayes Agnew—once a member of the Philadelphia General Hospital's staff—supports Croskey, with the laconic statement that the Almshouse was "the oldest hospital on this continent." Both doctors overlook the obvious primacy of Spanish and Frensh hospitals, to the north and south of Anglo-America; but much more significant to this study, they both claim hospital primacy for their institution, over the Pennsylvania Hospital.[32]

Proponents of the primacy of the Pennsylvania Hospital, however, are numerous and have had their day. They begin with Franklin, who noted in 1751 that "sick and distempered strangers" were provided a place of accommodation by the Assembly, and hoped that the Assembly would show "an equal tender concern for the inhabitants." Franklin obviously was referring to the Pest House, on Fisher's Island, as the place where "sick and distempered strangers" were being housed. Of greater consequence, is Franklin's desire that the "inhabitants" who were also ill, have a place of their own to go. Obviously, if the Almshouse was a real hospital, the "inhabitants" would have had such a place. Later champions of the Pennsylvania Hospital pointed out that the title, "hospital" was not even used to officially designate the medical branch of the Philadelphia Almshouse until 1836, and that the Almshouse sent many of its sick residents to the Pennsylvania Hospital for treatment, during the eighteenth centry. Those patients were paid for by the Almshouse, causing one champion of the hospital to note that had a hospital,

> "in connection with the Almshouse existed, the Guardians of the Almshouse would not have made an arrangement for the Managers of the Pennsylvania Hospital to take their curable sick paupers as pay patients, thus increasing the expenses of the Almshouse."[33]

Actually, the question of historical primacy is a problem of definition. It is only logical to assume that the Almshouse, from its very beginning, did attempt to heal its sick inmates, and may well have employed doctors for that purpose. As early as 1751, for example, Dr. William Shippen, Sr., was receiving a salary from the Almshouse. But curing the sick was only a corollary of the real function of the Almshouse. To shelter and feed the indigent was the primary purpose of that institution. It was not until the late eighteenth, and early nineteenth century, that the Philadelphia General Hospital could make a legitimate claim to being a "modern" hospital. By contrast, the Pennsylvania Hospital, from its inception in 1751, was primarily concerned with healing, and therefore, deserves to be called the first "modern" hospital in Anglo-America.[34]

By the mid-1760's, the old Almshouse on Third Street was incapable of meeting the needs of Philadelphia's rapidly growing population, and the Board of Managers of the Hospital sent an address to the Assembly, asking that some further provision be made, to deal with those newly discharged Hospital patients, who were yet too weak

> "to perform hard labor, and at a loss for the means of subsistence, till they recover their strength."

By 1767, on a site only one block west of the Hospital, a new structure was completed, which replaced the old Almshouse. This new structure was thereafter known as the Almshouse, or Bettering House and, or, House of Employment. Its function was to house and feed the indigent, and to provide work for those who were able, as well as to take care of "women in labor [the Almshouse probably did develop the first Anglo-American obstetrical clinic], and people with venereal diseases, and it also . . . [served] as a place of confinement for vagabonds, wrong doers and prostitutes."[35]

Perhaps inspired by the successful example of the Pennsylvania Hospital, the Assembly created a corporation, headed by twelve managers, to run the "new" Almshouse. Although it received some tax support, the new corporation was also dependent on charitable contributions. The new Almshouse was largely of Quaker inspiration, and on its board of managers were such Quaker Hospital Managers as Joseph Fox, William Masters, Hugh Roberts and Samuel Rhoads. Although relations between the two institutions were understandably amiable during the remainder of the colonial period, no "working" relationships were established.

During the American Revolution, the state legislature's suspicion of Pennsylvania Quakers, led to the exclusion of Quaker managers from the board of the Almshouse. The Supreme Executive Council of Pennsylvania may well have been moving towards the same treatment of the Hospital's Quaker Managers, in the spring of 1779, when it questioned the legality of the Hospital Board's election.

The new managers of the Almshouse evidently did an unsatisfactory job and, in 1788,

"the legislative assembly, having received a report from the inspectors of charitable institutions on the abuses which had arisen in their management, concluded that the best way to effect a reform would be to entrust this asylum [Almshouse] once more to the Quakers."

Quaker direction then began to bring order and improved somewhat the financial stability of the Almshouse.[36]

While the Revolutionary War was on, the managers of the Almshouse proposed that the Hospital take some of the Almshouse's sick paupers. The proposal was first made in 1781, and from that date, the Almshouse often sent some of its sick inmates to the Pennsylvania Hospital, at a constantly adjusted charge, per patient. The Hospital maintained that it charged the Almshouse no more for those patients than it cost the Hospital to shelter, feed and clothe them. The Almshouse, however, often declined to pay its bills, claiming that the charge per patient was too high, or that the Almshouse's financial position was quite desperate. Finally, in 1789, the Almshouse agreed "to an amicable suit" which might allow the Hospital to collect the money owed to it. The issue in the suit concerned residents of Pennsylvania who had been sent from the Almshouse to the Hospital. The Almshouse claimed that the Hospital should not charge for any poor patients from Pennsylvania, and thus, had no right to collect on Pennsylvania residents sent to it by the Almshouse. The suit ended in 1791, with a judgement in favor of the Hospital, and the Almshouse was forced to pay that institution, back debts amounting to £1,014 and "interest thereon, from the 12 of February, 1791, and the

cost of the suit . . ." This judgement also reaffirmed that the Hospital
had the sole prerogative to set its own admission policies.[37]

Having won its case, the Hospital turned around, some eight years
later (1799), and offered six free beds to patients from the Almshouse,
if the usual security for clothing and burial expenses were given. There
was, however, a stipulation involved; the Hospital insisted that its physicians choose the six patients to be admitted. The managers of the Almshouse

> "acceded to the proposition with great satisfaction and delight, because they
> apprehended from the nature of . . . [the Hospital] the maniacs would be the
> first part of the selection."

But the Hospital's physicians rejected the "maniacs," and insisted,
instead, on admitting cases that could be taken care of—according to the
Almshouse managers— by the Almshouse. Thoroughly upset by the Hospital physicians' actions, the Almshouse managers rejected "what they
at first conceived to be a generous overture. . . .". The Almshouse did
say, however, that it would reconsider its rejection, if only one half of
the six patients admitted to the Hospital would be

> "the three maniacs who are at present peculiarly troublesome, and very unfit
> inmates for this institution . . ."

The Hospital's Board reacted by suggesting that the two institutions
each appoint a committee, to meet jointly, in order to deal with the mis-
understanding. The Hospital hoped that, out of the committee meetings,
would come

> "a more perfect understanding . . . of the uses and designs of the two
> institutions than at present exists. . . ."

Apparently the Hospital's aim was to eliminate duplication of effort with
the Almshouse. In the Hospital's view, there was to be only one preëmi-
nent hospital in Philadelphia, and that one would be the Pennsylvania
Hospital.

The Almshouse had other thoughts, and expressed them clearly to
the state legislature in 1804. After disarmingly stating that they "would
wish to evade any invidious reflection . . ." on the Pennsylvania Hospital,
the managers of the Almshouse pulled no punches. The Hospital was
"shut against the poor" and "contains no more than sixty to eighty patients" at a time, and was therefore

> "not a very important adjoint to the medical school [University of Pennsyl-
> vania] affording few examples of disease and but limited lessons in practice
> to the students. . . ."

By contrast, the memorialists went on, the Almshouse "might be, in
this respect, rendered more eminently useful and instructive." It already
housed "an extensive hospital" and sufficient financial aid from the state
would, the memorialists implied, make the Almshouse the leading hospital in Philadelphia.[38] A rivalry begun in the late eighteen century,

seemed to be accelerating during the first decade of the nineteenth century, as Philadelphia's two leading charitable corporations exhibited all too human characteristics. Eventually, of course, the Philadelphia General Hospital, whose roots were in the Almshouse hospital spoken of by the petition in 1804, would surpass the Pennsylvania Hospital in size.

In Retrospect

With the dawning of the nineteenth century, Samuel Coates must have often thought back to some of the events of the Hospital's first half century. Perhaps he lingered on the marble steps leading up to the center building, first gazing at the pilasters, which drew his eyes upwards to the third floor. That was where the operating amphitheatre would be, once the interior was completed. "How Thomas Bond would have liked that room for his clinical lectures." Glancing back through the front gate on Pine Street, Coates' eyes would have been met by much the same rural setting viewed by Benjamin Franklin, when the plot on Eighth and Pine was first examined, as a possible site for the new Hospital. In his musings, Coates probably heard the voices of Uncle John Reynell and fiery Israel Pemberton, plotting their next move against the Proprietors, or perhaps he saw again, a gathering of the remnant Board, as it worriedly met to voice concern over the exile to Virginia of four of its members, during the Revolution.

By comparison, how politically uninvolved, at present, the Hospital seemed to be. Oh, it was true that Coates had little use for Jefferson's partisans—he called them "Demi-rats"—and probably most of the remainder of the Board had similar Federalist leanings, but partisan political intrigue and complications seemed to be a matter of the past, as far as the Hospital was concerned. While the legislature did not approve the last request for financial aid, this probably was indicative of a new laissez-faire attitude by the state government towards private charitable institutions in general, rather than a partisan vendetta against the Pennsylvnia Hospital. Indeed, the Almshouse would have a similar request for aid refused, a few years later.[39]

Whatever, Samuel Coates must have felt a swelling of unQuakerish pride, as he surveyed how far the Hospital had progressed since those dark years of the Revolution. To be sure, his greatest expectation had not been met—the Hospital's financial position was less sound than in those halcyon days prior to the Revolution—but neither had his greatest fears been realized. The Pennsylvania Hospital now stood, solid and symmetrical, a legacy of fifty years of Quaker managerial skill, and a monument to the social concerns of eighteenth century Philadelphia.

Chapter 6
Healing During the Recovery Years, 1784-1801

The Physicians

IN *Rebels and Gentlemen: Philadelphia in the Age of Franklin,* Carl Bridenbaugh points out that the presence of Benjamin Franklin in colonial Philadelphia, has led to a preoccupation with the life and character of colonial America's greatest citizen, at the cost of overlooking other Philadelphians, who deserve our attention. So, too, in dealing with the medical staff of the Pennsylvania Hospital, from 1784 to 1801, there is a similar danger. Ten physicians served the Hospital during this period, but the nonpareil Benjamin Rush, eighteenth century America's greatest physician, threatens to push the other nine into undeserved obscurity. And yet, a check of some of the available indices, points up the fact that Rush was in good company. The *Dictionary of American Biography,* even with its bias towards politicians, lists seven of the other nine physicians, as do Henry Simpson's *Lives of Eminent Philadelphians* and the *Dictionary of American Medical Biography.*

Among Rush's strong supporting cast were John Jones, author of the first book on surgery written in the United States; Philip Syng Physick, who earned the sobriquet "Father of American Surgery;" Benjamin Smith Barton, not only an outstanding physician, but one of America's foremost botanists; and Caspar Wistar, author of the first American text on anatomy. Indeed, by comparison with the Board of Managers, the physicians of this period seemed to be much more eminent men. Whereas, 80 percent of the physicians are listed in the *Dictionary of American Biography,* only 6 percent of the Managers achieved the same distinction. This is somewhat in contrast to the colonial period, when 22 percent of the Board, and 45 percent of the physicians, were significant enough to be listed in the *Dictionary of American Biography.* In short, the caliber of the Hospital's physicians, initially very high, according to eighteenth century standards, further improved with the approach of the nineteenth century.[1]

Among the ten physicians who served the Hospital during the recovery period, the influence of Edinburgh was even greater than in previous years. Nine of the ten had crossed the Atlantic to pursue their medical education, with London, Paris, Gottingen, Rheims and Upsala appearing on their itineraries. Looming above all the other stops in these medical odysseys, however, was the University of Edinburgh's medical school.

Five of the nine Hospital physicians who crossed the Atlantic, received their M.D. degrees from Edinburgh, while three of the other four, spent spent some time there taking courses. Even James Hutchinson, the lone physician who crossed the Atlantic, without making the pilgrimage to Edinburgh, and John Foulke, the only physician to limit his education to this side of the Atlantic, were not untouched by Edinburgh. The medical school faculty of the College of Philadelphia, where both Hutchinson and Foulke received medical degrees (bachelor of medicine), was predominantly Edinburgh educated.[2]

Just as in the colonial and revolutionary periods, many of the physicians were of a different political leaning than the Managers. Whereas such leading Managers as Samuel Coates and Robert Waln were staunch Federalists, Doctors Hutchinson and Rush were of the Jeffersonian persuasion. Indeed, so active in politics was James Hutchinson that, according to some Philadelphia Quakers, his death in 1793 "saved the United States from a total revolution."[3] Nevertheless, most of the other physicians and Managers did not play leading roles in the political struggles of the late eighteenth century, and there is little evidence that friction, caused by differing poltical persuasions, created any serious disharmony during the recovery years.

The physicians continued to arrange their schedules, so that a two-man team of doctors attended the Hospital twice each week, for a period of four months. Attendance, according to this schedule, was insisted upon by the Board, and only twice, during the months of January, 1786, and February, 1798, did the Board register any complaint on this score. But the Board did show its displeasure over other actions taken by some of the physicians. In 1798, the Managers complained of "several persons" who had been admitted by the physicians who,

"at the time of their admission appeared to be near their end and have died shortly after they were taken in. . . ."

Two years later, Doctors Parke and Barton were admonished for allowing another terminal patient to enter the Hospital. Earlier that same year, insane patient William Sharpe used a fork to stab another patient, and then turned on the nurse of the woman's ward, inflicting three or four wounds with the same instrument. Thomas Parke promptly prescribed continued freedom for Sharpe, to walk the halls and the yard of the Hospital. The Board criticized Parke's actions as dangerous, and ordered the steward to recommit Sharpe to his room.[4]

Much more alarming than the oversight of Doctors Barton and Parke, was a significant error of judgement made by Dr. John Foulke, in August of 1793. Philadelphia was reeling from a yellow fever epidemic and most Philadelphians, unaware that yellow fever was spread by a mosquito, thought that the dreaded disease was contagious. Because a special hospital (Bush Hill) had been set up for the victims of yellow fever, and because its own regulations stipulated that sufferers of contagious diseases could not be admitted, the Pennsylvania Hospital felt under no obligation to admit victims of the fever. Indeed, admission of even one case of the disease, represented an extraordinary threat to the lives of everyone housed at Eighth and Pine. Therefore, when two yellow fever cases were admitted by Doctor Foulke, the Board became very alarmed. The first carrier of the dreaded epidemic died almost immediately upon admission, but the second continued to live and was quarantined, after the Board demanded that Foulke

> "visit the said patient and . . . do everything in his power to prevent the increase of his disorder in the family."[5]

The Board's directive to Foulke was credited with preventing the spread of the epidemic inside the walls of the Hospital.

Following the initial outbreak of yellow fever in 1793, it returned to Philadelphia during the summer and fall of 1794–1796, 1798–1799, and periodically, over the next decade. During those perilous times, the Hospital's policy of excluding yellow fever patients continued, so it seemed, to be paying dividends, as there were no further outbreaks among the patients at Eighth and Pine.

With the outbreak of the yellow fever epidemic in Philadelphia, the Hospital's physicians were put to the test. Most of the more affluent Philadelphians fled the city to avoid contracting the fever, but some of the Hospital's physicians remained at their posts. In the late summer and fall of 1793, with yellow fever taking a tremendous toll—approximately 22 percent of those Philadelphians, who remained in the city, fell victim to the scourge—Benjamin Rush and Thomas Parke remained at their Hospital posts while James Hutchinson, although not on duty at the Hospital, performed vigorously among the general populace, only to contract yellow fever and die on September 6, 1793.

Not all of the Hospital's physicians were equally courageous about remaining in Philadelphia. By October, Doctors Shippen, Kuhn and Foulke had fled to the country, to escape exposure along with about half of the Hospital's Board of Managers.[6] But then, Doctors Shippen, Kuhn and Foulke were not scheduled for duty at Eighth and Pine that fall, and the Hospital, therefore, was not adversely affected by their absence. Evidently, during other outbreaks of yellow fever, the Hospital's scheduled attending physicians continued the tradition of remaining at their posts.

Overall, despite some of the above mentioned instances, relations between the Hospital's Managers and physicians were usually quite cordial. Physicians were often consulted on administrative decisions, and the two groups even seemed to enjoy each other's company, on occasion. Samuel Coates and Philip Syng Physick, for example, were good friends. In fact, Board-physician relationships were probably much more cordial than physician-physician relationships.

Benjamin Rush was the focal point for much of the acrimony among the physicians. At various times in his career, the dogmatic Rush crossed scalpels with Adam Kuhn, Caspar Wistar and William Shippen, Jr.[7] But perhaps some of the ill feeling generated by those disputes was, in the end, beneficial to the Hospital. Rivalry among physicians led to accusations and backbiting, but also must have contributed to increased efforts by individual physicians, in the hope of being less vulnerable to criticism by professional rivals.

The Medical Library

One way to protect a reputation was to expand one's knowledge of medicine. To this point, a growing Hospital library was invaluable. From 1774 to 1786, only four volumes were added to the library, although one of these was Edinburgh Professor William Cullen's two volume *First Laws of the Practice of Physic* (more evidence of Edinburgh's influence). The physicians were concerned about the failure to buy more books for the library, and recommended to the Board that more books be imported. In the next three years, £266 were expended, which was about four times the entire sum spent on books, prior to 1787.

Thanks to continued purchasing, the zeal of Dr. Thomas Parke and Samuel Coates, the guidance of London Quaker physician John Coakley Lettsom, and the considerable bequest of one hundred forty-two volumes from Sarah Zane in 1800; by 1801 the Hospital could boast of a medical library of about 1,700 volumes, an increase of almost 1,200 volumes since 1790. Anxious that quality be commensurate with size, the Managers had contacted Doctor Lettsom, stating that all of the Hospital's physicians agreed that Lettsom should select the appropriate books for the Library. Lettsom responded with a broad spectrum of selections that included German, French and classical works, as well as the standard English volumes. The costs of these new library books continued to be offset by student fees, paid to the Hospital's physicians. Initially located in the Managers meeting room on the second floor of the east wing, the library was moved to the first floor of the center building, in November of 1800. Although the Managers could justifiably boast that their library housed the best medical collection in the nation, the Board wished to make other collections available to the physicians and, in 1799, purchased a share in the Library Company of Philadelphia.[8]

The Anatomical Museum

Also, of continuing educational significance, was the Hospital's anatomical museum. Formed around the nucleus of John Fothergill's gift to the Hospital, the museum's exhibits were enhanced by new additions, from time to time. During the recovery period, the most significant new addition was the anatomical preparations of Philadelphia surgeon and anatomist, Abraham Chovet, which the Hospital purchased in 1793. Such observers as John Adams and the Marquis de Chastellux had already praised the anatomical preparations (dried, injected and painted specimens) while John Morgan was highly impressed with Chovet's wax models. Unlike the Fothergill models, the Chovet collection is no longer extant, having been destroyed by fire in 1888.[9]

Medical Students

Certainly, the anatomical museum and the library were as important to the Hospital's medical students, as to its physicians. Students who were not fortunate enough to be under the tutelage of one of the Hospital's physicians, were charged a yearly fee—$5 after 1793—for a certificate that gave them the right to walk the wards, and use the library. All students, including those apprenticed to Hospital physicians, had to pay in order to use the museum. In 1791, the Hospital's physicians proposed that their apprentices have a "perpetual privilege" to use the library and observe cases in the Hospital. The Board, stating that such an opportunity for life, is more than equal the service the students were rendering the Hospital, rejected the physicians' proposal.[10] Although the majority of the pupils did not render extraordinary service to the Hospital, they did dress wounds and performed other, less demanding chores, under their preceptors' directions. For the most part, however, they merely attended and observed; they did little work for the Hospital, and received a certificate testifying only to their period of attendance.

In addition to the usual medical students, during much of the recovery period the Hospital housed at least one medical apprentice. The medical apprentice was committed to a Hospital residence of four or five years, and received, at the end of that period, a suit of clothes, and a certificate, if the Hospital was satisfied with his service. Prior to 1800, four medical students were apprenticed in this fashion. The attraction of such an apprenticeship was obvious; in addition to ward duty, the resident apprentice was expected to help with weekly or semi-weekly clinical lectures given by Philadelphia's leading physicians. In fact, so attractive was the Hospital to aspiring young physicians, that those who had neither the money for the admission certificate, nor qualified to be appointed resident apprentice, often turned to gate crashing.[11]

By the mid-1790's, a subtle change had taken place in the duties of the resident apprentice; he was now functioning as the Hospital's resident physician. During the yellow fever emergency of 1793, apprentice Edward Cutbush became "prescribing physician." Thomas Horsefield, who followed Cutbush as resident apprentice, was given sole responsibility for the Hospital's out-patients. The resident physician, already found in most British voluntary hospitals, was fast becoming a fixture, in the brick building on Eighth and Pine. Up to this point, however, most of the indentured apprentices were in the process of simultaneously getting their medical degree from the University of Pennsylvania Medical

School, and usually completed that degree about the time their indenture ran out.[12]

Although Thomas Bond died in 1784, clinical lectures as well as other presentations relating to medical education, continued to be given at Eighth and Pine, with many of the Hospital's physicians holding forth. The relationship with the medical school (the medical school of the College of Philadelphia was merged with the medical school of the University of Pennsylvania in 1791) was more informal, than during the late colonial period, when Bond's clinical lectures were a required course for a medical degree. But the fact that many of the Hospital's physicians were on the medical school faculty, meant that medical students often gathered at Eighth and Pine, to hear their preceptors lecture, and to walk the wards.

According to some of those preceptors, too many students were sitting in on their lectures and, in 1791, Benjamin Rush tried to change the situation. Rush proposed to the Managers that a room be provided

> especially to accommodate a few patients, who were proper subject for clinical lectures . . .

and

> that none but his own immediate pupils attend his said lectures at the time he holds them.

The Board, although "disposed to oblidge Doctor Rush . . ." were of the opinion

> that the pupils to whom a full privilege of attending the Hospital is once granted, can in no case be prevented . . .

from attending lectures in the House. Thus, the certificate that enabled the neophyte physician to walk the wards, and use the library, also was upheld as a ticket into any of the lectures given at the Hospital.[13]

The Apothecary

The first postwar apothecary, Nicholas Waters, served from 1784 to 1787. Like his immediate predecessors, he received only room and board the first year. In 1785, Waters asked for a salary, and the Board, evidently pleased with his work, granted him £50 per annum. Upon Waters' resignation in 1787, the Board rewarded his three years of service, by granting him the right to "free use of the books in the medical library, without limitation of time." In turn, Waters promised the Hospital that "when his leisure will admit . . ." he would "attend and assist the new apothecary gratis. . . ."

The Board, wishing to reduce costs, then decided that William Gardner, resident medical apprentice, would fill the role of resident apothecary. Other resident medical apprentices followed in the same position, until well into the nineteenth century.

In 1800, the apothecary's shop was moved from the two story outbuilding it had been in since 1769, to the first floor of the center building. The shelves of the new apothecary shop were stocked with drugs which, unlike those of the colonial period, came from American suppliers.[14]

The Steward and Matron

Only two stewards and four matrons served the Hospital from 1783–1801, and the Managers were more than satisfied with each one. Joseph and Deborah Henzey had been hired in 1780 to serve as steward and matron, respectively. The Board's approval of the Henzeys—particularly Joseph Henzey—has been previously mentioned. By 1783, the Henzeys were receiving a joint salary of £110 per year, the highest joint salary ever paid by the Hospital.

Evidently, Deborah Henzey gave birth to four children between 1780 and 1786, and this created an awkward situation for the Board. Since the matron, steward and family slept, and ate their meals in the Hospital, the costs of continuing the Henzeys under employment, mounted with the rapidly increasing appetites of their four young children. In 1786, the Board's Committee on Economy pointed out to Joseph Henzey, that in the past, the two previous stewards were charged £15 per year for the board of each of their children. Thus the committee recommended that the salary of the Henzeys be reduced to £75 per year. After discussing the matter with the steward, the Board granted the Henzeys a reduced salary of £80 per year, a most equitable settlement in view of the four children being boarded.[15]

In 1790, Deborah Henzey died and Mary Falconer replaced her as matron. The Board then reduced Joseph Henzey's salary to £60 per year. The steward and the new matron were both unhappy with their salaries—the actual amount offered Mary Falconer is not recorded—and let the Board know, in no uncertain terms. Evidently, the Board saw merit in their complaints and, in the fall of 1791, consented to pay Henzey £90 per year—he was asking for £100—and matron Falconer, £30 per year. Henzey continued his duties as steward until struck down by "palsy" in 1796. Due to poor health, Mary Falconer had resigned as matron the previous year, and Henzey's oldest daughter, Ann, filled in. But with her father ill, Ann Henzey turned her attentions exclusively to nursing her stricken father, and the Board turned to procuring a new matron, as well as a new steward.

Francis Higgins and his wife Hannah, after an inquiry by a committee as to "their abilities," were hired in 1796, as steward and matron, respectively at the annual salaries of £100 and £35. After serving well in their respective capacities, the Higginses resigned their positions, in order to embark for Ireland in 1803. On their ocean crossing, they carried a certificate affixed with the Hospital seal, expressing that institutions's satisfaction with their performance.[16]

Increasingly, as the nineteenth century approached, the steward was becoming more specialized, and therefore less medical, in his function. Prior to 1780, the steward often filled in as apothecary or vice versa, but after that date, no steward assumed the role of apothecary, nor did any of the apothecaries assume the role of steward. (Of course the apothecaries during the period 1787–1801, were medical apprentices, and therefore, had neither the time nor inclination, to take on any extra burdens.) What was happening, was that the office of steward was abandoning any medical pretensions whatsoever—three of the colonial stewards had called themselves doctor—in order to concentrate increasingly, on the twin responsibilities, of business manager and director of employees.

All routine expenditures for food, fuel, repairs, salaries, furniture and medical supplies were disbursed through the steward's office. The apothecary, ostensibly under the direction of the physicians, received money for his purchases of drugs, from the steward. Equally significant, was the steward's responsibility for personnel employed by the Hospital. Even the female employees, although initially the responsibility of the matron, ultimately, were under the direction of the steward. By 1801, the personnel under the steward's direction, amounted to nine employees residing in the Hospital, and a gardener, stableman, gate keeper, washerwoman and some part-time help, who commuted daily from their homes in order to work at Eighth and Pine.[17]

Cell Keepers

As the number of insane in the Hospital increased, (see Appendix) the office of cell keeper became increasingly significant. The Board, no doubt aware of this fact, tried to be more selective than in colonial times, in hiring cell keepers. And yet the turnover of cell keepers was as rapid as in previous years. For the period 1752 to 1775, some twenty-four years, the Hospital employed twenty different cell keepers. From 1784 to 1801, some seventeen years, the Hospital employed sixteen different cell keepers, which represented a turnover comparable to the earlier period. The performance of the two groups of cell keepers, however, seems to have differed significantly. Whereas, the colonial cell keepers were often drunk on the job, and a disturbing influence to the inmates, no such complaints were registered during the recovery years. With a dramatic increase in the number of insane patients in the late 1790's (the new west wing was opened in late 1796), the one cell keeper needed help. In 1797, the first assistant cell keeper was hired, at about one half of the cell keeper's salary (the cell keeper was receiving £3 per month), while a "nurse of the cells" had been hired by 1800.[18]

Nurses and Other Staff

The generalization that the eighteenth century nurse was more a servant, than a trained part of the medical team, was nowhere more true than in the Pennsylvania Hospital, from 1784 to 1801. So low were the standards for nursing, that many female employees, hired originally for other positions, often served as nurses. Elizabeth Truby was hired as house maid in 1796, only to be listed as nurse, the next year and then as maid again in 1799.

Elizabeth Brown, cowherd for the Hospital in 1788, later became assistant nurse; Catherine Burns and Ruth Carrigan, Hospital cooks, also became nurses; Ann Gillispey followed the same route as Burns and Carrigan, only to later return to cooking. It is quite evident that no special requirements or qualifications separated nurses from the rest of the female staff, during the recovery period.

And yet the job made its peculiar demands. Not only were the nurses doing the normal work expected of their breed, but a few were becoming specialists in "laying out" the bodies of dead patients, a chore that paid extra. Nurse Kitty Burns became particularly expert in this melancholy task, receiving between seven shillings and one pound per body. In some years, Kitty "layed out" more than twenty bodies. To nurse Burns and others, mortality at the Hospital had its compensations.

The nurses were helped in their varied tasks by assistant nurses. Jane Fennel was hired as the first assistant nurse in 1793, only to show her versatility (or was it lack of specific training?) by becoming house maid, and then washerwoman. Salaries for the assistant nurses amounted, on the average, to seven and one half shillings per week or exactly the amount received by many of the nurses. In terms of yearly wages, most of the nurses and their assistants, were receiving in the neighborhood of £20 per year, along with room and board. This was higher than the average nurse received in colonial times, but this increase can be explained as a product of the inflationary forces, that generally pushed up costs, during the 1790's. The effects of this general inflation can also be seen in the steward and cell keeper's salaries, which were considerably higher than the salaries of their colonial predecessors. Colonial stewards averaged £70 per year, plus room and board, while their counterparts from the period 1784–1801, averaged about £100 per year, plus room and board. Cell keepers of the colonial era, averaged about £20 per year, plus room and board, while their later counterparts, averaged about £36 per year, plus room and board.[19]

By 1800, the Hospital employed a nurse for each of the two sick wards (men's and women's), a nurse for venereal patients, who were housed in the former apothecary building, and a "nurse of the cells." At least two assistant nurses were also employed, but this does not, by any means, exhaust the list of female employees. One housemaid and one washerwoman were continuously at work and, by 1788, a cowherd was employed. The cattle had materialized because of decisions made in 1786, when the Managers moved in a number of directions to cut costs. One means of reducing costs, was to increase the productivity of the Hospital garden, and to build up a livestock herd. (During the colonial and Revolutionary periods a few milk cows had been main-tained.) During the colonial period little mention is made of a cook. For the 1784 to 1801 period, however, we do know that the cook was always a female, who often had a female assistant.

In all, then, by 1800, there were nine or ten full time female em-ployees at the Hospital, most of whom received room and board and salaries of about seven and one helf shillings per week. Some of the nurses received ten shillings per week, but these were usually women with long years of experience at the Hospital. Beginning nurses started at the identical wage received by the assistant nurses, maids and cooks. This salary equality further points up the fact that nursing in the Hospital did not, during the late eighteenth century, continue the trend of the colonial era, which saw nursing become the highest paid position, with the exception of matron, open to members of the weaker sex. If salary is any criteria—and it often is—the Hospital nurses of the late eighteenth century, were losing their elitist status acquired during colonial times, to a new, seemingly egalitarian policy of the Board, towards all of the female staff under the matron.[20]

Compared to the colonial era, turnover of nurses from 1784 to 1801, was not as high, and a number of nurses remained with the Hospital for long periods of employment. Kitty Burns, Ruth Little, Abigail Lay-ton and Eleanor Baxter, between them, put in an aggregate of twenty-four years in the Hospital's wards, while steady employment for two or three years, was not uncommon among the other nurses.

Long term stability was also characteristic of the house maids who, even after taking inflation into consideration, were better paid then their colonial precursors. By contrast with the nurses and maid, the cooks tended to be employed for only short duration—there were seventeen cooks in seventeen years—but no comparison can be made with their colonial counterparts, since records on the latter group are so fragmentary.

Perhaps many of the female employees remained with the Hospital for an extended period, because their husbands were also employed there. By 1796, the Hospital staff included seven salaried males, and there was a good chance that some of those males, particularly if they lived on the grounds, wished to find employment in the Hospital for their wives. Thus Ruth Little, Hannah Savage and Sarah Little, all wives of cell keepers, served as nurses concurrent with their husbands' tenures, while Rachel Price served as cook during her husband's stay as stable-man. For many female employees, the convenience of neither husband nor wife commuting elsewhere to work, and the luxury of a second income, no matter how small, made it difficult to leave the Hospital's service.[21]

The Philadelphia Dispensary

In 1786, the number of sick-poor seeking medical aid at Eighth and Pine lessened somewhat, thanks to the establishment of the Philadelphia

Dispensary. (In 1927, the Dispensary became affiliated with the Pennsylvania Hospital.) Some historians have observed that the Dispensary actually became a more valuable instrument than the Hospital, for healing the sick-poor in Philadelphia, because the Dispensary treated far more patients. In its first five years, for example, the Dispensary treated nearly 8,000 patients, while the Hospital, during the same period, probably treated less than one fourth that number.[22] In defense of the Hospital, it must be noted that while Hospital out-patients were of the same type, and received approximately the same care as the patients of the Dispensary—this included some home visitations by physicians—the Hospital's in-patients were in a different category. Their ailments were so serious, and their plight so desperate, that they could not remain at home. Because medical treatment of the Hospital's in-patients was much more expensive, time consuming, and skill demanding, than the medical aid offered at the Dispensary, a comparison of the effectiveness of the two institutions, based on the number of patients treated, is, at best, misleading.

Admission Policies

The Hospital was hard put to find room for all of the deserving poor, not because there was not enough physical space, but because there was not enough money to provide adequate food and services. By 1796, the financially hard pressed Board had adopted a policy of limiting the number of nonpaying resident patients, to thirty at one time, although additional emergency cases might be admitted. The procedure for application and admission, continued to follow the general pattern of the colonial period.

In 1798, the Managers wished to do away with the burial guarantee, or deposit requirement, demanded of all sick-poor patients. But, according to the Hospital charter, the Board had to receive the approval of the Contributors, and certain state officials, before such an important change could be implemented. Evidently the Board failed to get the needed approval, and the burial security requirement remained. The failure of the Managers to push through this reform, continued to force prospective poor patients to find patrons, friends, relatives or Hospital officials, willing to pledge the necessary burial security. By 1803, burial security had reached five dollars per person.[23]

By contrast with the great hospitals of London, where admissions were processed only once a week, the Pennsylvania Hospital continued the practice, inherited from colonial times, of admitting patients twice a week. In earlier times admission days tended to be Tuesday and Friday, but Moreau de St. Méry, after visiting the Hospital in the mid-1790's, noted that two Managers and two doctors

"come every Friday and Saturday at eleven o'clock in the morning to receive and discharge patients. . . ."[24]

While the number of out-patients averaged about 250 per year, the number of in-patients increased in an irregular pattern, from 106 in 1783, to 176 in 1801. The number of resident patients at a given time, reflected this irregular increase in admissions (see Appendix). In 1783 there was an average of forty patients in residence; some eighteen years later, the number had increased to eighty-five. But the latter figure was still far short of the one hundred plus patients, of the last decade of the colonial period. Because the number of poor patients was necessarily kept down, due to financial imperatives, the bulk of the increase in resident patients, was in the paying category (see Appendix). By January, 1801, there were almost twice as many paying patients, as poor patients in residence.

The percentage of insane patients also greatly increased during the recovery period. On a given date during the colonial period, the resident physically ill outnumbered the resident insane, by two to one. Thanks to the addition of the west wing, by January of 1801, resident insane patients now outnumbered the physically ill, by better than two to one (see Appendix).[25]

Although most of the Hospital's beds were occupied by the insane, paradoxically enough the physically ill, because they usually remained for a much shorter time, represented the majority of patients admitted. Indeed, during the recovery years, the latter outnumbered the insane by better than two to one.[26] But admission statistics are not a faithful reflection of where the energies of the Hospital were focused. As the resident figures indicate, most of the beds, most of the time, were occupied by the insane, and this is clearly indicative of where the Hospital's energies were now concentrated. The shift in the nature of the Hospital, begun during the Revolution, continued during the recovery years.

Patient Care and Conditions

While most of the area around the Hospital remained bucolic right up to the turn of the century, this did not insure tranquility for the patients. That Philadelphia sport of viewing and baiting insane patients, begun during the colonial years, continued into the early nineteenth century. The practice of charging to view the patients, also begun in the colonial years, was continued by the Managers, with the admission fee set at about half a shilling during much of the recovery period.

Again, just as in the colonial period, these curious and sadistic visitors created problems. In 1784 the Hospital's physicians

"recommended that some regulations may be made in respect to persons visiting the Hospital, particularly in adopting such rules as would tend to prevent the lunatic patients from being interrupted and disturbed in their course of medicine."

The Board responded by adopting the rule that no more than two persons at a time

"be permitted to go into the cells and those persons to be attended by the cell keeper, and not suffered to speak to such patients."

This restriction was not enough to prevent continued disturbance of the insane and, in 1791, a new restriction insisted that visitors be approved by one of the Managers, physicians or the steward, before the cell keeper should let them in the gates.[27]

While curious and sadistic visitors continually interrupted and disturbed the insane, the insane, in turn, exercised a disturbing influence on the other patients. With only fifteen cells available for the insane prior to 1796, many "lunatics" had to be accommodated in the two sick wards. This led not only to disturbances but also to the danger of bodily harm to the other patients.[28] When, in December of 1796, the "lunatics" were removed to the newly built west wing, the increase in tranquility within the east wing, must have been considerable.

Noise was not the only complaint concerning conditions within the Hospital. The cells for the insane continued to be subject to dampness and cold. But it was common knowledge that the insane were not affected by temperature extremes! Evidently the Board took exception to this "common knowledge" because, by 1788, stoves had been installed in the basement "between every two cells." On November 11, 1789, Benjamin Rush, finding the stoves inadequate, informed the Managers that the cells, in which the insane were housed, "rendered abortive" any therapy he attempted. The winter cold, Rush went on, caused most of the cell occupants to catch

> "cold in two or three weeks after their confinement, and several had died of consumption in consequence of this cold."

The Board seems to have heeded Rush's lament, and charcoal burning stoves were placed in the basement. This proved an unsatisfactory solution because of

> "the great inconvenience to the health of the patients being apparent from the burning of charcoal . . ."

The board then charged the building committee

> "to devise a plan by which the cells may be safely and properly warmed by the burning of wood instead of charcoal in stoves and otherwise."

Because wood burning stoves could not safely be placed inside the individual cells, it is doubtful that a successful solution to this heating problem was reached, until well into the nineteenth century.[29]

In 1789, the Pennsylvania Hospital, along with a number of other institutions, petitioned the legislature for aid in procuring a water supply. Out of this initiative came the Philadelphia Waterworks, which began delivering water from the Schuylkill, to Philadelphia in 1801. But it was probably sometime after that date, before the Hospital possessed any but the most rudimentary water supply. Waterclosets were a thing of the future. As late as 1810, Benjamin Rush complained of the chamber pots used in the Hospital's cells, because of the noxious odors from the stools "discharged" therein. Moreover, chamberpots had broken while being used, causing, in the case of one patient, loss of life "in consequence of a wound upon the buttock. . . ."

Body wastes and garbage were buried on the grounds and attracted rats. Insane patient David Gibson complained vigorously of the "House Ratz," which "ran over" his face in the dead of night, and threatened to eat him, as well as his meat and bread. Gibson went on, in a slightly maniacal tone, about the threat to the world posed by the increasing rat population; but then, if one were restricted to a rat infested cell, the rodent threat could assume outlandish proportions.[30]

Again, cleanliness and sanitation were judged by the standards of the day, and judgement of visitors to the Hospital seems to be generally favorable for the period 1784 to 1801. The few negative reports seemed to have centered on the basement cells of the eastern wing. In 1797, with the insane now housed in the new western wing, Liancourt commented on the cleanliness of the new cells, and the overall economy, of the insane section of the Hospital. Nevertheless, "two years since," that section "was a subject of disgust." Almost nine years earlier, Benjamin Rush had complained of the "offensive and unwholesome" odor in the cells, and proposed more wholesome apartments be provided.[31]

Among visitors favorably impressed by conditions in the Hospital, was Brissot de Warville who, in 1788, found cleanliness "everywhere" and noted that each cell contained "a large window with bars and shutters opening on a yard." A year earlier, Manasseh Cutler found the cells to contain either beds or "clean straw", and everything "about" the insane patients, "was neat and clean." Cutler was so taken by the Pennsylvania Hospital, that he wrote that the institution at Eighth and Pine "seemed more like a palace than a hospital, and one would almost be tempted to be sick, if they could be so well provided for."

During at least part of this period, hot and cold baths existed in a nearby building, but were used primarily for therapy, as most Philadelphians rarely bathed, or even admitted to the necessity of such activity. The necessity of cropping patients' hair, was viewed in a different light, however. Barbers were hired to cut hair and shave the patients, sometimes as often as twice a week. In view of the omnipresent vermin, the latter action is understandable.[32]

Just as with the colonial years, observations on the diet of the patients is seriously hampered because only a few diet schedules, for the eighteenth century, are extant. By examining the steward's cash books, however, enough information can be assembled to make some generalizations. Gruel (a thin porridge) made of corn or rice for breakfast, mush or flour pudding, and sometimes meat for dinner, and broth and beer for supper, formed the substance of the daily diet. In addition eggs, cheese, butter, chocolate, a large variety of vegetables, some fruits (apples, limes) and some seafoods (clams, oysters, and fish) were added to the diet, depending on the season, and the Hospital's financial situation. A daily ration of bread, either "soft" or biscuit," was also alloted each patient.

Meat seemed particularly a problem, as it was sometimes rancid on delivery. In 1786, an angry Board ordered the steward to cancel a contract with a local butcher, because "the provisions he furnished [were] not . . . wholesome. . . ." To insure itself of a supply of fresh meat, the Hospital, as previously mentioned, raised its own livestock. In 1790, steward Joseph Henzey reported that four calves, six hogs and two shoats had been slaughtered from the Hospital's own herds. Meanwhile the Hospital's garden was expanded and produced wheat, as well as vegetables. In a move linked to the recommendations of the Board's Committee on Economy, a baker was hired, part time, to bake bread "at the House." Although an economy measure, it also insured fresh bread for the patients.[33]

By comparison to contemporary British hospitals, the Pennsylvania Hospital fed its patients at least as well. Since much of the food was produced on the grounds, the diet of a patient at Eighth and Pine must have featured, in season, more fresh produce and meat, than the diet offered to many of his British counterparts. Nevertheless, the British Hospital's tendency to serve gruel at breakfast, meat or cheese for dinner, and bread and beer at supper, was imitated at the Pennsylvania Hospital. For the seriously ill patient on both sides of the Atlantic, there continued to be a number of special diets, which were probably more debilitating than health restoring. The fact that, now more than ever before, the Pennsylvania Hospital wished to attract many paying patients, was an added inducement to keep meals up to a certain minimum standard.[34]

Increasing Quaker antipathy towards "strong drink" after the Revolution, buttressed by the medical observations of Benjamin Rush, served to place restraints on the amount of alcohol served the patients at Eighth and Pine. In view of this attitude towards liquor, in 1786 the Board's Committee on Economy was startled to uncover the fact that

> "in 1785 upon an average four times more wine is charged than was in 1773-1775, and fifty percent more of rum, although the patients in 1785 were not half the number."

Obviously, much of the alcohol was being used by cell keepers and nurses, to pacify and tranquilize patients who were unruly, or in pain. After that date, Hospital records show a definite decline in the amount of liquor purchased up until 1792, when a very large consignment of alcohol was delivered. However, wines rather than rum and other "hard" liquors, made up the bulk of this shipment.[35]

Even more than in colonial times, when Thomas Bond handled most of the surgery, and probably most of the insane cases, the physicians turned to specialization. James Hutchinson, until his death in 1793, and then Caspar Wistar and Philip Syng Physick performed most of the surgery. While Hutchinson, Wistar and Physick rarely made incisions into the skull, thorax or abdomen of their patients—antisepsis was still far in the future, and therefore this sort of operation usually proved fatal—they did amputate appendages and extract wens (tumors), stones, cataracts, and repair aneurisms and hernias.[36] Functioning primarily in the capacity of physicians, as the eighteenth century understood that term (diagnosticians who prescribed cures but left surgery to the surgeons), were the remaining doctors. This did not mean, however, that some minor surgery could not be performed by the other physicians.

Although, in 1753, Morgagni maintained that pathology was a matter of anatomy, and therefore focused attention on specific diseased areas of the body, those who subscribed to the various "systems", continued to dominate American and British medicine. The University of Edinburgh was particularly attracted to a "systematic" approach to pathology, which maintained that there was one cause for all diseases. This systematic approach left its imprint on the young American medical students, who later served the Pennsylvania Hospital. Particularly affected, was Benjamin Rush, who first adopted the systems of Edinburgh medical school professor William Cullen, and then that of Cullen's pupil, John Brown. Finally, Rush opted for a "system" of his own, that viewed all disease as a matter of vascular tension, which could be best remedied, by removing great quantities of blood.[37]

Phlebotomy (bleeding) had long been practiced at the Hospital, but probably not to the degree sought by Rush. Again, because the physicians' record book is not extant, we do not know exactly what therapy was administered in the Hospital during the eighteenth century, but there is other evidence to support the view, that, during the colonial period, therapy was less drastic than that later advocated during the recovery period, by Rush and some others.[38]

Rush was a very persuasive exponent of phlebotomy, and by 1795 had converted the very capable Philip Syng Physick to his views. Rush's "system" and its resultant therapy (copious bleeding) was not, however, accepted by some of the Hospital's physicians. James Hutchinson, mortally ill with yellow fever, refused Rush's pleas for copious bleeding and purging. Others did not wait until they were on their death beds, to take exception with Rush. Adam Kuhn and Caspar Wistar openly criticized Rush's therapeutic methods (this criticism went beyond bleeding as it also questioned Rush's practice of administering strong purgatives). It must have given Rush a great deal of satisfaction when, during the yellow fever epidemic of 1795, he reported to a friend that

> "Kuhn and Wistar have been forced to retreat to our remedies, and the disease under the depleting treatment, properly extended, has become less mortal even in their hands."[39]

Because some of the other Hospital physicians did not agree with Rush's extreme methods, this did not mean that their diagnostic findings and theraputic prescriptions, were correct by modern standards. A patient with physical problems was fortunate in having Adam Kuhn, rather than Benjamin Rush, not because Kuhn's diagnosis and treatment were more in line with modern medicine, but because Kuhn was less committed to a "system" and therefore less given to extreme or heroic measures.

When Thomas Bond resigned from the Hospital in 1784, no one physician seems to have taken over responsibility for the insane. In 1787, however, all doubt as to who would direct the care of the insane ended, when Benjamin Rush "obtained exclusive control of maniacal patients."[40] Rush retained this position into the nineteenth century and, because he was in charge of the insane patients, and because the insane represented more than one half of the resident patients, at a given time, it is incumbent to examine Rush's therapeutic approach to insanity.

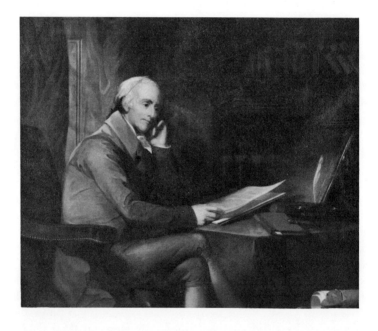

Rush had a genuine committment to aiding the insane, but just as in the case of his predecessor, Thomas Bond, Rush's committment took an ironic twist when, in 1810, his son John was admitted to the Hospital, suffering from "the disease of the mind." Moreover, one unconfirmed source maintained that beautiful Polly Hefferman, an insane patient at the Hospital, had been, prior to her illness, the focus of Rush's romantic interests. While at the Hospital, Polly succeeded in locking Doctor Hutchinson in her cell, and came perilously close to killing Doctor Parke, when her knife thrust "pierced through his coat and jacket, and plugged from the wall behind him, a triangular piece of mortar."[41]

Unfortunately, Rush's empathy for the insane was not matched by a "modern" diagnosis of mental illness. To Rush, "madness" was mainly a vascular problem, having its primary seat in the blood vessels of the brain. "Madness" was caused by an inflamation, or morbid excitement of the brain, by too much blood. Since excess blood flow to the brain was the cause, the remedy was obvious: blood flow to the head must be slowed, and the total amount of blood in the body, reduced. Thus, just as in physical maladies, copious bleeding was often called for, but extensive phlebotomy was not the only therapy to be used. In 1787, Rush wrote Doctor Lettsom, in London that in his work with the insane at the Hospital, "the remedies on which I place my chief dependence, are warm and cold baths." Perhaps, typical of Rush's therapy at the Hospital, was the "bleeding . . . strong purges, low diet, kind treatment and the cold baths," administered to fourteen cases of "mania" in 1796. The purpose was, quite clearly, to decrease or redirect the flow of blood in the body. In terms of modern therapy, Rush's system seems wrong headed; but to observers of his day, there could be no denying that a violently insane patient, tended to calm down under the debilitating effects of bleeding, purging, limited diet and cold-water shock treatments. It is no wonder that, when Warville visited the Hospital in 1788, the staff informed the Frenchman that none of the insane were violent.[42]

Warville also noticed that insane patients were dealt with much more humanely, in the Pennsylvania Hospital, than in France. The great French reformer, Philippe Pinel, would introduce dramatic changes in the treatment of the insane, in his country, but not until the next decade. The increasingly humane way that the insane were treated at the Pennsylvania Hospital may, in part, be attributed to Quaker concern for these unfortunates (Was it just by chance that England's great reformer in this field, William Tuke, was a Quaker?), and the energetic efforts of Benjamin Rush.[43] In his attempt to have the Hospital's insane treated more humanely, Rush adumbrated some of the reforms introduced by Pinel and Tuke. Rush constantly complained, as previously noted, about the dampness and cold in the cells, and the need for better accomodations. Once the insane had been moved to the new west wing, in late 1796, Rush turned to other means of granting some dignity, to the lives led inside those new cells. He proposed that

> "certain employments . . . be devised for such of the deranged people as are capable of working."

This, of course, was not an innovation, but rather renewed emphasis on an old Hospital practice, going back to 1754. Later Rush attacked the use of the "madshirt," or straight jacket, used to confine the violently insane.[44]

Despite the efforts of Benjamin Rush and a sympathetic Board, it was not until 1796, that living conditions for the insane in the Hospital, even foreshadowed modern standards. In 1795, for example, the Managers were

> "oblidged, in some instances, to confine more than one lunatic in the same apartment [cell] . . ."

Rush may later have argued against the use of straight jackets, but they were centainly in use through 1801, as were chains and other restrictive devices. By contrast, by 1801, Bicêtre in France, and the York Retreat, in England had done away with chains, and treated their patients as "guests." Even the debilitating therapy, practiced by Rush, was greatly moderated in the case of Bicêtre, or completely discarded, in the case of the York Retreat.

Rush's work with the Hospital's insane was not without its apologists, and foremost among them was Rush himself. For the ten year period 1793 to 1802, Rush claimed to have cured 174 patients and to have relieved 101 others. Samuel Coates, who should have known as much as any Manager about the patients of the Hospital, lent support to Rush's claims by noting, in 1796, the amazing recovery made by some lunatics. Coates went on to say that

> even yesterday when I was at the Hospital, a man was discharged entirely well . . . [and] no man could appear more distracted than he did ten days ago.[45]

To summarize the therapy administered in the Pennsylvania Hospital during the recovery period, is to summarize the therapy administered by Benjamin Rush—after all, all of the insane after 1787, and many of the physically ill from 1784 to 1801, were his responsibility—and add that the treatment administered by the other Hospital physicians, differed from Rush's, only in degree. The same bleeding and purging that Rush used to heal his patients, was followed by the likes of Kuhn and Wistar, but in more moderate portions.

A Look at the Record

While Rush and his colleagues would put great stress on the number of patients who were discharged as cured, again mortality statistics offer an alternative way to evaluate the Hospital's performance. For the years 1783 to 1802, some 3,408 resident patients were treated in the Hospital, and some 458 died. This represented a mortality rate of 13 percent, which was slightly higher than the mortality rate for the entire colonial period, but significantly an improvement over the mortality rate for the Revolutionary War years. The slight increase in the mortality rate, over that of the colonial period, may reflect the failure of the more humane measures introduced by Rush and others, to completely compensate for Rush's addiction to "heroic" therapy.[46]

Chapter 7

The Abdication of Leadership: 1801-1841

WHETHER in its territory, population, industry and commerce, or in the size of its institutions, nineteenth century America was characterized by extraordinary growth. From 1801 to 1841, Philadelphia and the Pennsylvania Hospital reflected this national growth trend and yet, by 1841, both the Quaker City and the Hospital had lost their former positions of preeminence. New York, not Philadelphia, was now the largest and most important urban center in the nation, while large municipal and state hospitals were attracting more attention, and caring for more patients, than the Pennsylvania Hospital. During the late eighteenth, and early nineteenth centuries, the example of the Pennsylvania Hospital served as inspiration to the founders of a number of hospitals including, in particular, the New York, and Massachusetts General.[1] However, by the second quarter of the nineteenth century, the Philadelphia institution, in a reversal of roles, was emulating the examples set in Boston and New York.

Although Philadelphia did not grow as rapidly as a number of other American urban centers, its growth was, nevertheless, nothing short of spectacular. Urban Philadelphia's population shot upwards from about 68,000 in 1800, to about 232,000 in 1840.[2] As in Colonial times, the number of sick-poor endemic to the Philadelphia area was augmented, particularly during and after the 1830's, by a large number of immigrants. In addition to the great increase in the number of poor suffering from somatic illnesses, the number of insane, from all levels of society, seemed to be increasing even more rapidly than the population as a whole. It is against this background that the Pennsylvania Hospital searched for a new role. Once the archetypal American general hospital, the brick structure at Eighth and Pine could no longer consider itself the forerunner of the American hospital of the future. Because government subsidies had ended with the passing of the eighteenth century, the Pennsylvania Hospital just did not have the resources to offer succor to large numbers of sick-poor. Rather, it was in the area of experimentation, and in the popularizing of new methods and techniques in treating patients, and in the training of physicians, that the Pennsylvania Hospital would have to carve out its particular niche in American social and medical history, during the years 1801 to 1841.

Government Aid and Tax Exemption

The attitude of the Pennsylvania legislature was particularly vexing. During the eighteenth century, the legislature had repeatedly voted financial assistance to the Hospital, for construction programs, and to build up the depleted capital stock. The legislative grant of 1796, however, marked the end of direct public assistance until the twentieth century. It wasn't that the Hospital didn't try to raise funds from the reluctant legislators. Indeed, in addition to direct requests for aid, the Hospital worked hard at good public relations with the Pennsylvania Assembly, by continuing to submit annual reports, and by giving each member of that bicameral body, a copy of the official history of the Hospital, published in 1831.[3] The refusal of the Pennsylvania Assembly to grant financial aid, must have been particularly frustrating when, only 83 miles to the northeast, the New York Hospital continued to receive considerable state aid throughout the first half of the nineteenth century.[4]

Even more upsetting than the state's unwillingness to render financial aid, was the attempt by the city, county, and eventually the federal government, to tax the Hospital, and the reluctance of the state legislature to intercede on the Hospital's behalf. In 1808, the city and county of Philadelphia, assessed the Hospital for the first time in the Hospital's history.

The Board's refusal to pay the tax, caused the tax collector to seize some of the Hospital's cows and hay. Repeated requests to the state legislature, for an act exempting the Hospital from taxation proved futile, and the Hospital was left with no alternative but to pay its taxes. A prior dispute between the Hospital and the Guardians of the Poor of Philadelphia, over rates to be charged mental patients sent to the Hospital by the Guardians, probably alienated some influential members of local and state government, and created in both levels of government, a certain lack of sympathy for the Hospital's plight.

In 1814, the situation took on an even more ominous turn, when the U.S. Congress made ready to pass a bill that would place a federal tax on all property, taxed by county governments. Since the Hospital now fell into that category, its tax burden was bound to double. The Board pointed this out to the Assembly, but it wasn't until 1816, after the Hospital had paid a year's federal tax, that a public petition convinced the state legislators to grant the Hospital tax exemption. The tax exempt status of the Hospital was further clarified by an act of the state legislature in 1845.[5]

The Board of Managers

While struggling to maintain its tax exempt status, the Hospital's attention was also focused on a number of other problems. Very simply put, the Hospital found itself caught between the pressing need to specialize, and expand its physical facilities, and the reluctance of the state government to financially support these changes. The responsibility for finding a way out of this conundrum fell, of course, to the Board of Managers.

As in previous years, the Board continued to show a heavy Quaker representation, with 49 percent of the Managers who served from 1801–1841, of the Friendly persuasion. Of those who served five years or more, 50 percent were Quakers. Moreover, during this period, the three presidents and the three treasurers, were Friends. Indeed, so powerful an influence did those of the Friendly persuasion continue to exercise over the Hospital, that Dr. George B. Wood felt compelled to argue, in 1851, that the Pennsylvania Hospital was not now, or ever had been, governed exclusively by Friends.[6]

Mercantile interests continued to be the most representative vocation among the Managers, but the dynamic economic changes sweeping the nation were also reflected in the activities of some of the Board members. Thomas P. Cope, for example, was very prominent in the import-export business, but eventually found himself much involved in the Chesapeake and Delaware Canal, and in the Pennsylvania Railroad, while Mordecai Lewis moved from mercantile pursuits, to factory ownership.

Board members were very active in other philanthropic organizations with prison reform, charity schools, food for the poor, and the development of a public school system, taking up much of their time and energy. There didn't seem to be any specific type of charity favored over all of the others. Roberts Vaux, for example, worked hard to establish a public school system, so that the poor could develop the tools to help themselves while, at the same time, participating in food handouts to paupers.[7]

And yet there is no doubt that the Board wished the Hospital to be a particular type of charity; that is, above all else, to continue the tradition of the Hospital's earlier years by aiding, in particular, the "deserving" sick-poor. The will of Board president Josiah Hewes, the admission policies adopted for the new lying-in department, and random comments in the Board's Minutes, all indicate that good character and industriousness continued to be desirable traits, and were rewarded accordingly, when decisions were made on which applicants would be admitted as poor (nonpaying) patients. Indeed, the emphasis on serving the deserving poor, was so all pervasive at Eighth and Pine, that even Morton and Woodbury in their *History of the Pennsylvania Hospital,* published in 1896, used the term "deserving poor persons."

Of course, Philadelphia's tremendous population growth made it impossible for the Managers to personally know the overwhelming majority of applicants for admission. Although recommendations from other Philadelphians, or other Pennsylvanians of some standing in their respective communities, might partially fill this void, it is probable that admissions of sick-poor patients, due to the difficulty of establishing whether they were "deserving" or not, was probably less selective than in the eighteenth century.

But there can be no question as to the intentions of the Managers. In 1817, by some oversight in the admission procedure, an unmarried female was admitted into the lying-in department. An angered Board immediately resolved that in the future

> "no person be admitted to the benefit of that department unless satisfactory evidence be produced of her living in lawful wedlock, and that she did so at the period of her becoming pregnant."

Pennsylvania Hospital physician John Redman Coxe summed up the philosophy of the Board, when he described a truly useful philanthropic institution, as one that performed

> "the greatest good with the least means. . . . The relief granted should hold forth no temptation to increase the number of those applying for it, or in the most distant way to encourage vice or idleness, . . ."[8]

Although not quite as distinguished in its membership as the colonial Board, the Managers of the early nineteenth century were often men of considerable influence and wealth. Alexander Elmslie left the very sizable estate, for that day, of some $400,000 to his heirs; Samuel Coates was a director of the First Bank of the U.S., Roberts Vaux declined a similar appointment to the Second Bank of the U.S., and Joseph Watson was mayor of Philadelphia for three years.[9]

Raising Money

Without government aid, the Board's management of, and solicitations for, the capital stock took on added significance. That the Board met with some success is indicated by the growth of the capital stock from $58,000 in 1801 to more than $260,000 by 1833. Contributions to the fund for the new hospital for the insane, were so combined with the capital stock after 1833, that the two could not be separated until 1843, by which time the capital stock had reached $310,000 (see Appendix).

The traditional method of conjuring up philanthropic impulses, by publishing Hospital histories, produced separate volumes in 1801, 1817, and 1831. Unlike the eighteenth century, however, there were no sudden increases in contributions, immediately after publication. By far the largest individual benefactor of the Hospital, was merchant-banker Stephen Girard, whose first wife had died an insane patient, at the Hospital in 1815. Between 1786 and 1816, Girard contributed over $4,000 and, in 1832, the Hospital received an additional $29,250 from Girard's will. John Keeble, another wealthy Philadelphian, left a legacy of land, which the Hospital sold off in individual parcels for approximately $27,000 between the years 1808 and 1851.[10]

While Philadelphia's merchant princes continued to render considerable financial support to the Hospital, such people as attorney Horace Binney, coach-maker Robert Fielding, carpenter James Greeves, milkman George Branner, and even teacher Ann Saunders also contributed respectable sums. As in previous years, contributors were not limited to this side of the Atlantic. Robert Barclay, of London, continued his financial support right up to 1816, and new support came from the likes of Dublin printer Philip Whitfield Harvey.[11]

Benjamin West

One of the most important contributions from Great Britain, came in the form of an oil canvas, produced by the Pennsylvania expatriate Benjamin West. In 1800, at the urging of Samuel Coates, the Board sent a request to West in London, asking for the donation of a painting. West accepted the request and proposed to undertake a ten by sixteen feet painting of Christ, healing the blind and lame, in the temple. The Board approved the subject matter and promised to exhibit the painting in the Contributors' room in the center building. In turn, West promised that his canvas would be completed by the spring of 1803.

Unfortunately for the Hospital, West did not make good on his promised completion date. In early 1804, Samuel Coates' son, John, wrote his father from London that, after dining with West, the painter assured him that the work would be completed during the next summer. The painting was already on its frame, the outlines drawn, and the subject completed in miniature. The younger Coates noted, however, that although West was exceedingly industrious, "he would probably be more expeditious if some appeal were made to his vanity."[12]

Five years went by and still no painting! Again the younger Coates met with West and this time was told that, although the painting was not yet finished, it was of such great consequence that it should be donated to the state of Pennsylvania, as well as to the Hospital. John Coates, no doubt angered by the artist's delaying tactics and puffed up self esteem, and certainly no admirer of the Pennsylvania Assembly, argued with West that the state legislature had little interest in art and, furthermore, was disposed to encroach on Hospital privileges, and might even go so far as to claim the painting for itself. Evidently, John Coates was convincing because West agreed to forgo his "favorite project of dignyfying his present." Coates relayed to his father, West's promise to send the painting to Philadelphia by next August, but added that West now expected the Hospital to supply the frame.

With the canvas almost in his grasp, Samuel Coates wrote the celebrated artist, of his joy that "the most valuable painting that was ever presented to this country, or perhaps to any part of the world . . ." would soon be on exhibit, at the Hospital. West's poor health further delayed the completion, but in 1810 West apologized and pledged to resume work, as soon as his health permitted. It was with astonishment, that the Managers next heard that the work was completed, but that West had been persuaded, through the payment of 3,000 guineas, and entreaties from a number of influential Englishmen, including the Prince of Wales, to sell the painting, so that it might be used to start a national gallery in England. West did promise, however, that he would produce a copy for the Hospital, that would be a little different from the first painting, thus creating an original.[13]

Initially very perplexed with West's actions, Samuel Coates and his fellow Managers felt a good deal better when reports reached them of the acclaim accorded West's recently finished work, and the willingness of large crowds to pay for the right to see the painting. Joshua Gilpin wrote from London, that by selling the first painting of Christ healing the lame and blind, West had increased the value of his eventual gift to the Hospital, ten fold. Moreover, the exhibition of the painting had already produced £9,000 sterling! Not leaving anything to chance, however, Samuel Coates continued to remind, cajole and flatter West.

The War of 1812 may have interrupted West's concentration, but in 1814, the expatriate painter requested a separate room in the Hospital, for the exhibition of his soon to be completed masterpiece. West seemed irate when it was reported to him that some Philadelphians were making uncomplementary remarks about the sale of his first painting, which had been promised to the Hospital.

In 1815, after hearing that the Hospital had agreed to erect an exhibition building to display his painting, West announced that the canvas was finally finished. Thanks, in part, to special contributions from such private benefactors as Stephen Girard, the Hospital made ready a small brick structure, facing Spruce Street, which contained a large upstairs exhibition room for West's painting and a basement room for the museum collection. West was displeased with the reported Gothic appearance of the building—West, after all, was a product of the Enlightenment, and had little use for things medieval—but in October of 1817, the painting arrived in Philadelphia with the suggestion from West, which was approved by the Board, that the viewing fee be $.25 per person. On West's request, painter Thomas Sully, who had already done portraits of Samuel Coates and Benjamin Rush for display at the Hospital, helped with the placing of the painting in the exhibition room, and then co-authored a pamphlet on the work.[14]

The Managers were very pleased with West's painting, referring to it as "a precious performance." In November, the first viewers were admitted, and by the end of 1841, almost $20,000 had been added to the Hospital's coffers, from fees paid for viewing the painting. Perhaps even more important than the added income, was the fact that large numbers of Pennsylvanians and others, were becoming, for the first time, familiar with the Hospital. In the first twelve months that West's canvas was on display, better than 30,000 people rode or walked out to the Hospital to see it.[15]

What exactly were those hordes of people paying to see? Christ healing the lame and blind in the temple can be viewed today on the

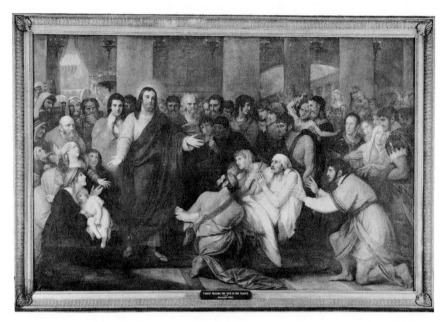

back wall of the entrance foyer of the Hospital's administration building, facing Eighth Street.

To this twientieth century viewer, the painting hardly rates the encomiums lavished on the canvas, almost a century and a half ago. Massive in size, it somehow lacks the human dimension, because it is wanting in the warmth and passion, that such a scene should conjure up. In short, West's important gift to the Hospital is a product of eighteenth century restraints, that somehow make the work less than appealing, although it does retain a certain compelling historical significance.

Other Sources of Income

Much more important in fiscal terms than West's painting, was the annual income, generated by the growing capital stock. Increasingly, as the nineteenth century developed, the Hospital moved away from investing in ground rentals. Back in 1801, about 50 percent of the invested capital stock had found its way into ground rentals, but by 1841, that figure was down to about 5 percent. By the latter date, mortgages and personal notes represented over 90 percent of the invested capital stock, with securities, such as bank stocks, representing the remainder.[16]

In 1798, Congress embarked upon a health insurance program of sorts, by authorizing deductions from the wages of seamen, to be paid to the collectors of customs who, in turn, were to spend the money, under the direction of the President of the U.S., for the relief of sick and disabled seamen. The mode of relief depended upon the individual seaport. In the Boston area, where there wasn't as yet a hospital, a marine hospital was built in Charlestown. Providence and Newport simply boarded afflicted seamen in private homes, while in New York and Philadelphia, where there were hospitals, a contract arrangement was set up, whereby the collector of customs paid a specified rate to the hospitals, for each admitted seaman.

Although the occupations of the patients, admitted to the brick building at Eighth and Pine were not systematically recorded, the type of injury, or an occasional note of a specific patient, indicates that almost from the very inception of the Hospital, sailors were patients. In 1800, the Hospital agreed with the collector of customs for Philadelphia, to admit U.S. seamen—evidently military, as well as civilian sailors were included—at $3.50 per week. This arrangement, with a few short interruptions, continued down to 1880. The arrangement was not, however, without some rancor. One particular issue was the length of time, some seamen were spending in the Hospital. The U.S. government's position was, that relief was to be "temporary and not be be extended to incurables. . . ." The Hospital's position was, that since the government was paying the bill, albeit after collecting from the sailors, the Hospital could well afford to be more charitable than usual, and allow these particular patients to remain for indefinate periods. The fact that it probably made a small profit on each admitted seaman, may have influenced the Hospital's attitude.

In 1807, customs collector Peter Muhlenberg stated that he would not be security—that is to provide for clothes and burial expenses if necessary—for any seaman who stayed beyond six months, but the Hospital responded that it would not receive pay patients "under any limitations of time." In 1809, Muhlenberg's successor, John Steele, demanded that all seaman being paid for by the U.S. government be discharged. Benjamin Rush responded that some of the patients were in no condition to be removed. Evidently, the exchange put an end to this particular dispute, but other disagreements followed, focusing on the issue of how much per seaman, the Hospital was charging.[17]

Lying-In Department

In 1793, the Pennsylvania Assembly authorized the Hospital to establish a lying-in and foundling department, but this time the legislature found the Hospital dragging its feet. A foundling department was thought really outside the purpose of the Hospital, and, as for taking in pregnant women, there was some feeling that this too wasn't the proper role of the Hospital. Although Dr. William Shippen, Jr., had done much to advertise the value of obstetrics, in Philadelphia in the 1760's, it still wasn't accepted practice in many quarters, that a physician should be present at childbirth. To some, it was considered improper, and even indelicate, for an expectant mother to be attended by a male. Moreover, it was argued, wouldn't the Hospital's acceptance of poor, expecting mothers be an encouragement to vice and immorality? To those Managers who were not turned against the legislature's proposal, by the above arguments, there was the problem of limited finances, which precluded any attempt to found a lying-in department in 1793.[18]

Influenced by developments in Great Britain, a lying-in hospital was opened in New York City in 1799, only to be absorbed, two years later, by the New York Hospital. In Philadelphia, in 1802, a lying-in ward was opened in the Almshouse. Therefore, by December of 1802, when Samuel Coates proposed to his fellow Managers, that a lying-in department be established at Eighth and Pine, he was simply advocating that the Pennsylvania Hospital follow the examples already pioneered by two other American institutions.

With the Hospital in better financial shape than in 1793, and the new building program just about completed, both the Managers and the physicians, wholeheartedly concurred with Coates' proposal. The lying-in department was opened on the second floor of the east wing in May, 1803. Four years later, the First City Troop of Calvary of Philadelphia, turned over, for the use of the lying-in department, shares in the Bank of Pennsylvania, received from the U.S. government, for services rendered during the Revolution. The donation amounted to a capital of $6,400 and yielded an annual income of $456.50.[19]

In 1810, Dr. Thomas Chalkley James was appointed the first "physician to the lying-in department." Already a physician to the Hospital, James had also been instrumental in the founding of the lying-in ward, at the Almshouse. In 1817, several deaths from puerperal fever, occurred in the lying-in department, and James pointed an accusing finger at the "offensive effluvia", rising from the fracture ward, located just below the lying-in department. Following the recommendations of James and three of the other physicians, the Board moved the lying-in department down to the Contributor's room, in the first floor of the center building.

In 1824, the lying-in department was moved to what is now the historical library; but six years later, fever again broke out, claiming two lives and causing the removal of the remaining maternity patients, to the southwestern room, on the second floor of the west wing. The move was to no avail, however, as puerperal fever struck again, claiming two more lives. Acting on the advice of the two attending Managers, the Board then closed down the lying-in department, only to open it the next year, after Dr. James deemed it safe. Again, in 1835, puerperal fever broke out, and the lying-in department was moved to the bottom floor of the picture house. Further outbreaks of fever led to the abandonment of the lying-in department in 1854.[20]

Out-Patients

The Hospital's out-patient department, was established during the eighteenth century to aid, in particular, those suffering from "contagious or infectious" diseases and, therefore, ineligible for Hospital admission. Occasionally, Hospital physicians or apprentices would go out and actually visit the sick-poor in their homes. In 1807, this practice was formalized, as one physician was assigned the responsibility of the Northern Liberties, and another, the Southwark section of the city. Out-patient care never seemed totally satisfactory to the Managers, and that department was constantly being reorganized, with particular attention to avoiding interference with the practices of the Philadelphia Dispensary. The out-patient department was administered separately from the rest of the Hospital and, by 1809, out-patient physicians were drawing a salary of about $300.00 per year. In 1817, because the city established new dispensaries for out-patients, in the Northern Liberties and in Southwark, it was decided to shut down the out-patient department. Although only fragmentary records exist of out-patient care at the Hospital prior to 1797, over 16,000 out-patients were treated in the next twenty years.[21]

Relations With Other Institutions

Relations with other institutions took up much of the Board's time. Disagreements with the Almshouse during the late eighteenth and early nineteenth centuries, have already been mentioned. What was particularly bothersome to the Almshouse, was the fact that, while it paid to have its sick inmates treated at the Pennsylvania Hospital, other sick-poor who were recommended by the Guardians of the Poor for Philadelphia County, were often admitted as non-paying patients. But even the Guardians of the Poor were not completely happy with this arrangement, because they did provide clothing and burial expenses, for the patients they recommended while the "whole credit results to the Managers of the Hospital." Relations with the Almshouse and the Guardians of the Poor, seemed to improve after the War of 1812, and by 1815, medical apprentices of the Almshouse and the Pennsylvania Hospital, were allowed to view operations performed in either institution.[22]

The University of Pennsylvania had a history of formal and informal relations with the Hospital, dating back to the founding of the former institution's medical school, in 1765. During the last decade of the colonial period, the clinical course conducted at the Hospital by Thomas Bond, had been a requirement for a medical degree, at the College of Philadelphia, the progenitor of the University of Pennsylvania. Although an informal relationship between the two institutions continued through the late eighteenth and early nineteenth centuries, the University of Pennsylvania decided, in 1817, that a formal clinical course, taught at the Hospital by one of its medical school professors, would be very advantageous. The medical school's proposal to the Hospital, called for two separate wards, one male and the other female, to be set up exclusively for the use of the clinical instructor. Each ward was to accommodate at least fifteen patients, and would be provided with nursing care by the Hospital staff. The clinical instructor was also to have a "portion of the maniacal and venereal disease patients" under his care. Although the Managers recognized the significance of the proposal for advancing medical knowledge and training, they rejected the University's overture, because the proposition would have infringed on the rights of the Hospital's physicians.

The rejection of the University's proposal did not interfere with good relations between the two institutions. In 1824, the Hospital sent its museum collection to the medical school, because the collection would be "rendered more useful to the interests of science under the management of the University." The University, in turn, invited the Managers, physicians and surgeons of the Hospital, to join in the commencement procession of the medical school in 1825, and nine years later, the University donated a number of books to the Hospital's library.[23]

An Internal Disagreement

In 1825, Samuel Coates' failing eyesight forced him to step down as president of the Board. Over the forty-one years that he served as a Manager, Coates exerted a moderating influence on his colleagues. As if to point up this fact, in a little more than two years after his resignation, the Board was convulsed with the most bitter disagreement in its history. Back in 1786, with the Hospital trying desperately to pull itself out of the financial crisis brought on by the Revolution, the Board had established the Committee on Economy, to help the Hospital live within its limited income. Samuel Coates was a key member of that committee which, over the years, acquired increasing power over personnel, as well as over the other internal operations of the Hospital. In 1824, the Board appointed the Board of Female Assistants, to regularly visit the Hospital, to offer advice to Hospital employees, and

> "to report from time to time to the Managers individually or collectively such alterations and improvements in the internal economy of the House as they may judge salutary, useful or needful."

Samuel Coates' second wife, Amy Horner Coates, seemed to exercise a great deal of influence on the Board of Female Assistants, and, initially, the actions of this female advisory body met with Board approval.[24]

In December, 1827, the Board of Female Assistants told the Managers of "their united disapprobation," of retaining operating room nurse Sarah Malin "in the Hospital in any capacity whatever." Evidently the Committee on Economy had already demanded the dismissal of Sarah Malin—the charges were never spelled out—but the matron and steward did not concur. This led to a showdown at the next Board meeting, with Manager Charles Roberts proposing that the Committee on Economy be abolished, but the twelve-man Board split down the middle on Roberts' proposal. Roberts then moved that responsibility for hiring and firing servants and nurses, be the steward's prerogative, "with advice of the attending Managers." Obviously, if Roberts couldn't abolish the Committee on Economy, he would try to strip it of much of its power. The Board adopted Roberts' second proposal, by a vote of eight to four, and some three months later, formalized the end of the Committee on Economy and the Board of Female Assistants; but not before the resignation of the entire Board of Female Assistants and five disgruntled Managers, with the latter explaining "that under the existing circumstances we can render you no acceptable or efficient aid." The remnant Board then nominated five Contributors to fill the vacant Board seats, and exonerated Sarah Malin from the charges made against her.[25]

Constructing a New Building for the Insane

The most important Board decision during the period 1801–1841, was to separate the insane from the somatically ill, by moving the former to newly constructed buildings, in West Philadelphia. The moral treatment of the insane, practiced at Bicêtre, in France and the York Retreat in England, was also becoming popular at Eighth and Pine. One of the essential constituents of the moral treatment, was the adoption of an efficient system of classification and employment. Unfortunately, the crowded and restricted facility at Eighth and Pine, made an efficient system of classification and employment of the insane, almost impossible. Moreover, some of the residents living near the Hospital, were beginning to complain of the noise and commotion created by the insane.[26]

In 1831, the Managers spoke wistfully, of procuring building funds so that the insane could be provided with adequate space. After deciding to lay the problem of the acute shortage of space squarely before the Contributors, the Board proposed to the Contributors, that a separate asylum be set up for the insane. Since the Hospital had continued the process begun in the eighteenth century, of purchasing nearby lots, it was decided that some of those lots might be sold off in order to raise funds to build an additional building.

A disagreement then developed over a Board proposal to separate the physically ill from the insane, by building a separate structure to house the physically ill, on the block directly south of the Eighth and Pine building. The Board even went so far as to solicit architectural drawings for the proposed structure. But at a Contributors meeting, Philadelphia attorney, Horace Binney strongly advocated that the insane department be "removed from the city of Philadelphia to the country in its vicinity. . . ." The Contributors went on record in favor of Binney's proposal, even though the Board felt "that an insane hospital can best be managed within the limits of the city." After hearing Manager Charles Roberts strongly advocate the Contributors' viewpoint, the rest of the Board grudgingly gave in, and laid before the Contributors, a general plan for a separate insane hospital that "should not be beyond four miles from the city." The Contributors, after asking for some more details and some alterations in the building plans, directed the Managers to purchase a proper site.

In 1835 the Hospital paid $28,000 for Matthew Arrison's 101 acre farm, which was situated west of the Schuylkill River, in the general area of 44th and Market Streets. At the time, this site offered the bucolic setting that experts felt was necessary for the proper treatment of the insane. Three years later an additional 9½ acres was purchased for "walking grounds" for the patients. Despite the objections of gadfly Manager Charles Roberts, the Board decided to open a quarry on the newly purchased farm, to produce building stone for the new asylum. A handsome brick mansion, built in 1794, and a stable were to be left standing for the Hospital's later use.

With the approval of the Contributors, final plans were adopted and English architect Isaac Holden, who had come to this country in 1826, was chosen to design the new structure, after a contest in which at least two other leading Philadelphia architects—John Haviland and William Strickland—had entered drawings. Holden, who had previously acted in the capacity of consultant on the proposed asylum, drew up plans for a main building with a classical motif, capable of holding 170 patients

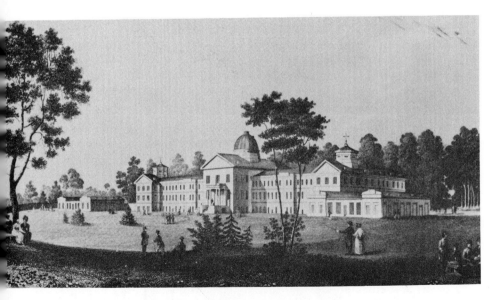

Pennsylvania Hospital for the Insane.

and numerous staff. The structure was not to be capable of indefinite extension, out of due regard to "architectural propriety."

While the main building was to house most of the insane, patients characterized as "furious and those of unclean habits," were to be housed separately. The idea of separating the most disturbing and unruly patients from the rest was a matter of common sense, as the Hospital's records were replete with complaints of violent and vocal insane patients, disturbing the tranquility of the others. Moreover, the desire to isolate the most troublesome patients, was reinforced by the knowledge that this practice was carried on elsewhere.

In 1838, Holden returned to England, leaving the direction and completion of the new asylum, in the hands of architect Samuel Sloan. The main building was completed at the cost of $165,000, and opened, for the transfer of the insane patients from Eighth and Pine, in 1841. Two detached buildings for the most difficult patients, male and female, respectively, were authorized in the same year and finished in 1842. In future years, the insane department would be called Kirkbride's, in honor of its first superintendent, Dr. Thomas S. Kirkbride.[27]

The Physicians and Surgeons

To be elected an attending physician to the Pennsylvania Hospital, continued to be a sought after honor during the first half of the nineteenth century. As one biographer of Philip Syng Physick pointed out, "his appointment to the hospital had a considerable influence in promoting his success, and leading to an extension of his business." Of the thirty-one attending physicians who served from 1801–1841, 74 percent are listed in the *Dictionary of American Medical Biography*, and 55 percent are included in the *Dictionary of American Biography*. The Board of Managers seems less distinguished for the same period, as only 10 percent of them are included in the *Dictionary of American Biography*.

Among the attending physicians, were some of the most honored names in the pantheon of American medical history. Continuing their service from the late eighteenth century, were Philip Syng Physick, Benjamin Smith Barton, William Shippen, Jr., Benjamin Rush and Caspar Wistar. Distinguished new additions to the staff, during the 1801–1841 period included Thomas Chalkley James, John Syng Dorsey, John Rhea Barton and John C. Otto.

The vast majority of the newly elected attending physicians, received their medical degrees from the University of Pennsylvania. European training also appeared on many vitae, but not as often as in the eighteenth century. If a Hospital physician had gone to Europe, London and Paris were more often on his itinerary than Edinburgh.

Specialization, a process followed increasingly in the larger American towns and cities during the early nineteenth century, had its impact at Eighth and Pine. The establishment of a lying-in department in 1803,

naturally led to the appointment of Thomas Chalkley James to the post
of physician in charge of that department, in 1810. In 1820, a second
physician, John Moore, was added to the staff of the lying-in department.
Others who served in that department prior to 1841, included Charles
Lukens, Hugh Hodge and Charles Meigs. Meigs, who often referred to
his patients as "dear little ladies," became a prime example of nineteenth
century male chauvinism, when he concluded that the female has "a head
almost too small for intellect but just big enough for love."

Since the very early days of the Hospital, surgery had been almost
the sole prerogative of the likes of Doctors Bond, Hutchinson, Wistar
and Physick. The Board, however, did not make an official distinction
between physicians and surgeons until 1821. After that date the attending staff generally included, in addition to the two physicians of the
lying-in department, three general physicians and three surgeons, with
the attending staff deciding on its own schedule of attendance.[28]

As the nineteenth century wore on, the attending physicians seemed
less inclined to impassioned political commitment, than did their predecessors. Gone were the likes of Benjamin Rush and James Hutchinson,
who were just as skilled at dashing off Jeffersonian polemics as they
were at cutting for the stone, or pleading for more humane care for the
insane. There were, as in previous years, occasional disagreements between the attending staff and the Managers. In 1801, for example, Doctor
Shippen was admonished for signing an admission form "without visiting
the said patient." Evidently the admitted patient was suffering from
yellow fever and soon died of the disease. The Managers were upset
because, like their eighteenth century predecessors, they believed that
yellow fever was contagious and, therefore, the admission of one case
of the dreaded disease, imperiled the entire patient population at Eighth
and Pine. The physicians made specific requests concerning the management of the Hospital, from time to time, but the Board often turned
down these requests only to reconsider them at a later date. For example,
the idea that the Hospital needed a salaried apothecary originated with
the physicians, only to be initially rejected and then, at a later date,
instituted by the Board.[29]

Medical Apprentices and Resident Physicians

The Hospital continued to depend on resident apprentices for protean
labors. Usually a junior and a senior apprentice simultaneously served
the Hospital, with the senior apprentice given most of the responsibility.
As in the later part of the previous century, the apprentices acted as
house physicians, apothecary, physicians to the out-patient department,
and even librarian. Upon leaving the Hospital, the apprentice would
often acquire additional experience and reputation, such as aboard a
foreign-bound ship, or at the Philadelphia Dispensary. If the young
physician went on to acquire a considerable reputation, he might even

be invited back to Eighth and Pine, as an attending physician or surgeon.

During the first two decades of the nineteenth century, the apprentice situation became somewhat confused, as degree holding physicians began to act as resident physicians, and physicians to the out-patient department. Sometimes these resident physicians were salaried, and might even take over the apothecary shop. But this arrangement varied according to the year, and it wasn't until 1824 that the Board implemented the policy of ending apprenticeships, and allowing only graduates with medical degrees in hand, to serve as resident physicians. After 1824, two resident physicians—one to take care of the insane and the other to handle the remaining patients—simultaneously served the Hospital. Usually a resident physician was a young man looking for more experience and, therefore, willing to perform services at the Hospital for a year or two, for room and board and little else.[30]

In all, these resident physicians represented an unusually capable group, with some of them eventually making notable contributions to the advancement of medicine. Included in this group were Thomas Kirkbride, who would be recognized as a national leader in the treatment of the insane; John Rhea Barton, who developed a new surgical technique for operating on the hip joint; and William W. Gerhard, who first identified typhoid as a distinct disease.

The Library

During the first two decades of the nineteenth century, an increasing number of medical students attended the Hospital. From 1804 to 1815 alone, some 1500 students, most of them fee-paying, received instruction at Eighth and Pine and this, in turn, meant a large increase in the library fund. In fact, during some years so much money was accumulated that some of it was spent on other Hospital programs. The most important single addition to the library during the early nineteenth century, was the acquisition of some 200 works on natural history, once owned by Benjamin Smith Barton and sold to the Hospital in 1817 by his widow for $2,770. Other purchases and gifts gradually increased the size of the library so that by 1830, despite numerous complaints of book thefts, there were some 5,828 volumes, and seven years later over 7,300 volumes. As late as 1850, a committee of the American Medical Association reported that the medical collection in the Hospital's library, was still the largest in the nation.

In 1807, the library was moved from the first floor of the center building, to the long room on the second floor of the same structure. The library remained in the long room—the present site of the historical library—until 1824 when it was moved, probably back to the first floor, to make way for the lying-in department. In 1835, with the lying-in department moving out to the Picture House, the library returned permanently to the long room. Responsibility for the library passed from the apprentices to the apothecary and, finally, to the newly created position of clerk of the Hospital.

Board interest and support for the library was led by the ubiquitious Samuel Coates, and later by Charles Roberts. Among the physicians, Thomas Parke was the strongest supporter of the library. This support was particularly appreciated, in face of a decline in student fees paid to the Hospital, during the third decade of the nineteenth century. Evidently this decline in student fees was attributable, in part, to the fact that many of the Hospital's physicians, such as Rush, Shippen, Wistar, Coxe and Dorsey, who were also professors at the University of Pennsylvania's medical school, had resigned their Hospital positions by 1820, thus making a trip out to Eighth and Pine, less attractive than formerly to students at the University. Another attraction to students, the Hospital's museum collection, had been loaned to the University in 1824.[31]

Medical Students

The decline in the number of students may have been lamented on the one hand, but it must have been a relief of sorts on the other. Full of youthful pranks, medical students continued to be a bane to hospital authorities throughout the Western World, during the early nineteenth century. In the previous century, medical students at the Pennsylvania Hospital, were accused of unruly behavior, unauthorized use of dead bodies, and numerous other transgressions of hospital etiquette. Complaints about the deportment of students at Eighth and Pine continued after the turn of the century, with specific complaints being leveled at students, for disturbing the insane patients in such a way as to "retard their recovery." Pupils were cautioned, continuously, about their behavior while in the Hospital, with the students of Doctors Shippen and Physick, particularly, subject to such warnings. The students of Shippen and Physick resented the warnings and wrote the Board, in 1806, that to the Managers, blackguards and medical students were synonymous. The Managers responded with an apology for casting aspersions on the character of the students, but also pointed out that some of the latter had not paid for the privilege of using the Hospital, and therefore, had no right to be in the building.[32]

The Apothecary

During the late eighteenth century, the financially hard pressed Hospital, had turned to using one of its medical apprentices as apothecary. But with the steady improvement of the Hospital's financial situation, thought was given to going back to the colonial practice of employing a professional apothecary. The physicians were insistant on this change, but the Board dragged its feet, despite numerous complaints about the functioning of the apothecary department. In 1808, Dr. P. C. Barton served briefly as a salaried apothecary, in addition to his other duties as resident physician and surgeon, but soon, medical apprentices were again preparing drugs and filling prescriptions for Hospital patients.

In 1820, because the cost of last year's medicines was "beyond all precedent," a committee of the Board undertook a detailed investigation of the apothecary shop. Among its negative findings, the committee cited the attending physicians' "reiterated complaints of the frequent absence and inattention of the apprentices. . . ." Although the committee went on to make a number of proposals to improve the administration of the apothecary shop, the physicians were not satisfied. But, when the latter again proposed that a professional apothecary be employed and an elaboratory be erected, the Board turned down both proposals. Some eleven months later, however, the Board had second thoughts on employing a professional druggist, and hired Graham Hoskins as apothecary and librarian. In 1823, Dr. Robert Harris replaced Hoskins, only to be fired, when an investigation found a great deal wrong with the apothecary shop. Samuel Sheppard served for a year and then resigned to be replaced by Newberry Smith, Jr., at the salary of $250.00 per annum, plus room and board. Four years later, Smith was succeeded by Franklin Smith, at $400.00 per year. Smith was replaced, in 1831, by John Conrad, who served as apothecary until 1870. Conrad, who was very well thought of by the Board and staff alike, went on to get his M.D. degree from Jefferson Medical College in 1850.[33]

The Steward and Matron

As the chief executive officer of the Hospital, the steward found his powers considerably enhanced by the demise of the Committee on Economy, in 1828. Over the previous years, the latter committee had usurped many of the prerogatives that, logically, should have been the steward's. After 1828, the steward and matron were again solely responsible for the hiring, firing and the direction of most of the Hospital's personnel. As in the previous century, the matron was usually the wife of the steward and functioned as his subordinate.

When Francis and Hannah Higgins sailed off to Ireland in 1803, they were succeeded as steward and matron, by William and Abigail Johnston, at the combined annual salary of $466.67 plus room and board. In 1807, the Johnstons resigned, without words of praise from the Board, and the Higginses, who were back from Ireland, consented to return to the Hospital. By 1812, the Higginses were making a combined salary of $600.00 per year plus room and board. The next year, the Hospital was saddened by the death of Francis Higgins, whose "long and faithful services . . . justly entitled him to the respect and confidence of the Managers."[34]

Samuel and Mary Mason made an excellent initial impression on the Board, and were subsequently hired at the same salary as the Higginses.

Some of their burden was lightened when the Board directed Samuel Mason to hire a husband-wife team, to act as director of the lunatic department, at the joint salary of $300.00 per year plus room and board. Within a year, the new directors of the lunatic department were fired by the Board and their positions were abolished.

The Masons seemed to have pleased the Board, as evidenced by periodic salary increases. Then, after some twelve years of employment, the Masons informed the Hospital of their impending resignation, which was to take effect in March, 1826. The standard scenario reads that those two well-loved Hospital administrators were highly praised as they left the Hospital for some other worthwhile pursuit. But it didn't work out that way. No words of praise are recorded as the last days of the Masons' employment drew to a close. Indeed, only a month after the couple left the Hospital, Manager Roberts Vaux asked that Samuel Mason's activities, while employed by the Hospital be investigated. It seems that Mason, on leaving the Hospital's employment, set up his own private hospital for insane patients, in the hope of turning a nice profit. In order to attract paying insane patients, already housed at Eighth and Pine, Mason spread stories among the friends and families of some of these patients, giving an "unfavorable opinion of their treatment and condition with a view to their removal from the Hospital to an establishment of his own. . . ." The controversy between the former steward and the Hospital seems to have been short lived, however, as no further mention is made in Board meetings, of Mason's private asylum.[35]

Isaac and Ann Bonsall were hired to replace the Masons, at $800.00 per year plus the usual room and board. Matron Bonsall's responsibilities were limited to the east wing of the Hospital, because the west wing was under the direction of Alice Harlan, who had served as the first matron of the lunatic department, since 1821. The creation of the latter position reflected the growing number of insane patients being housed at Eighth and Pine. In 1829, Harlan resigned, without being praised, and the Board promptly abolished her position which, in turn, left matron Bonsall with increased responsibilities. Evidently the matron handled the extra load in admirable fashion and took a particular interest in the insane. When Ann Bonsall died in 1830, at the age of fifty-eight, she was highly praised for her overall performance and, in particular, for her "kind and successful treatment of the insane."

Isaac Bonsell was also well thought of by the Board, although he did clash with resident physician, John Wilson Moore. By reading between the lines, one gets the feeling that young Doctor Moore, perhaps a bit overly impressed with himself, wasn't being treated with the requisite amount of respect, by the older steward. Whatever, Moore complained of Bonsall's conduct towards himself, only to have the Managers decide that this was a personal matter, that should be settled by the two involved. An irate Doctor Moore responded to the Board's decision by handing in his resignation.[36]

With the death of his wife, Bonsall suggested that the Board look for a new husband-wife combination to serve as steward and matron. The Board agreed, but did ask Bonsall to stay on until a suitable couple could be found. In October, 1830, after a three month search, Allan and Margaret Clapp were hired, and a highly praised Isaac Bonsall resigned the position that he held for four and one half years.

The Clapps were paid $1,000 per year plus the usual room and board. The Hospital was very pleased with the new steward and matron, and it was with a great deal of sadness that the Board noted the matron's death in 1835, after a painful and protracted illness. Contrary to previous practice, the steward remained at his job at $800.00 per year while Margaret Robinson was hired to fill the recently vacated matron's position at $200.00 per year. The new matron resigned after only one month and the Board directed Clapp to find another. Elizabeth Clapp was chosen—it is unclear what relation, if any, she was to the steward—and remained until 1842.

In 1833, in an unprecedented move, the Board appointed Clapp to one of its committees. This decision upgraded the position of steward to the point where the office was not only carrying out policy, but actually beginning to get involved, on the periphery to be sure, in policy making itself. In retrospect, Clapp's tenure marked a real watershed in the development of the Hospital's chief administrative position, and set the stage for further development of the steward's powers and responsibilities, under William Gunn Malin, who succeeded Clapp in 1849.[37]

The Clerk

Because of the increasing amounts of money being handled by the Hospital, in 1819 the Board decided to hire a salaried clerk to keep the books and accounts, and to attend the visitors to the Hospital. Pierce Butler was the first clerk, and served admirably until 1825 at $20.00 per month plus room and board. At Butler's resignation, William Gunn Malin, a Moravian and a recent immigrant from England, was hired. Along with Dr. Thomas Kirkbride, Malin was destined to be the outstanding Hospital administrator of the nineteenth century.

Malin continued as clerk until 1841, and then served as steward of the Hospital's insane asylum. Finally, he returned to Eighth and Pine as steward in 1849, and continued in that position until 1883. An extraordinarily amiable and courteous man, Malin was largely a self educated lover of books. Although his interests were not in the field of medical studies, Malin did show a great interest in the treatment of the insane. It was Malin, as clerk in 1828, who first presented the Board with the observation that it was necessary to provide a separate asylum for the insane. Six years later, Malin followed up this initial presentation with a paper on the employment of the insane.

Nor did Malin neglect to write on other aspects of the Hospital. In 1825, Malin was given the additional responsibility of librarian, and in 1829, he presented the Board with a catalogue of the library's collection, along with a sketch of the library's history. In 1831, Malin's *Some Account of the Pennsylvania Hospital; Its Origin, Objects and Present State,* was published by the Board. The Hospital rewarded Malin's outstanding service by continually increasing his salary so that by the mid 1830's, he was receiving $500.00 per year plus room and board.[38]

The Rest of the Staff

Information concerning the remainder of the staff during the early nineteenth century is difficult to come by. Because the number of staff had increased with the growing number of patients, very few references to individual employees are made in the Hospital's records. There aren't for example, many references to individual staff firings for drunkenness or insubordination, which often appeared in the Hospital's eighteenth century records. Generalizations, therefore, about the character and tenure of such employees as the cell keepers, or the nurses are impossible to make. What can be seen, however, is that the increased specialization practiced by the Hospital's physicians, was characteristic of the rest of the staff.

By 1831, four cell keepers and eight female attendants were employed to handle the insane. In addition, ten nurses and assistant nurses and four male attendants were assigned to the physically ill. The staff in charge of the physically ill, was further divided into such specialty areas as the operating room and surgical ward, and the venereal house. Although it wouldn't be until the second half of the nineteenth century that nurses would begin to receive formal instruction, one gets an intuitive feeling, that during the first half of the nineteenth century, the caliber and performance of the Hospital's nursing corps, was superior to that of its immediate predecessor.

As in previous years, male employees continued to draw a much higher salary than their female counterparts. But even among the female staff, contrary to late eighteenth century practices, a considerable distinction was made in salary, with the nurses being paid considerably more than the assistant nurses, maids and cooks. Because nurses were once again the highest paid and, with the exception of the matron, the elite of the female staff, they often remained with the Hospital for an extended period of time. Nurse Mary Early, for example, showed her devotion to the Hospital by giving a hearth rug to the library, after some forty years of employment at Eighth and Pine.

And yet, whether nurse, cook or cell keeper, the salary difference between the chief administrator and the rest of the staff was greater than today. Nurses, for example, received about $100.00 per year plus room and board while the steward received up to $800.00 per year plus room and board and, in the case of Dr. Kirkbride, the supervisor of the newly opened asylum in West Philadelphia, $3,000.00 per year.[39]

The Patients

Towards the end of 1840, the number of resident patients in the Hospital on a given date was up to 216, or three times the 1801 figure. The percentage of insane patients on a given date gradually decreased from 68 percent in 1801, to 47 percent in 1840. As in the eighteenth century, the insane, because they remained so much longer than other patients, represented a much smaller percentage of all of the patients, admitted during a given year. For the Hospital year ending in April of 1801, for example, only 27 percent of admitted patients were classified as insane, but that figure was an even lower 6 percent in 1840.

The ethnic nature of the patients at Eighth and Pine was also changing, with the Irish born representing about 38 percent of admitted patients during 1840. In terms of vocational pursuits, sailors were the most numerous. The heavy representation of sailors is understandable, in view of the agreement between the port collector and the Pennsylvania Hospital. Middle class Pennsylvanians continued to send relatives to the Hospital's insane department, while preferring to remain at home, for the treatment of somatic illnesses. Paying patients represented about 65 percent of resident patients at a given time in 1801, but as the Hospital's financial position improved, this figure decreased to 40 percent in 1840.[40]

With the insane assigned to the west wing, the Hospital engaged in further segregation of patients by relegating venereal cases to an outbuilding, which was the former apothecary shop (elaboratory). Because the venereal house was too small to accommodate the increasing number of patients, the Board decided to add another story in 1817. The Hospital continued to charge venereal paying patients more than the other physically ill paying patients. A case in point was Ebenezer Keys who was admitted, in 1832, as a venereal patient at $4.00 per week. But when his disease proved to be a "lumber abscess" instead, his board was reduced to $3.00 per week. In what was probably a departure from eighteenth century policy, the Hospital segregated blacks from whites. The Hospital also discriminated between Pennsylvanians and non-Pennsylvanians, by charging paying patients in the latter category an extra $1.00 per week. This discriminating policy towards non-residents of Pennsylvania, had been urged on the Hospital by the Philadelphia Almshouse, during the late eighteenth century. Although the Hospital sometimes denied it, the fee charged paying patients continued to produce a small profit, which helped pay for some of the nonpaying patients.[41]

Just as in the eighteenth century, there were three ways that the sick-poor could obtain admission. They could meet the criteria for admission as nonpaying patients, if there were empty beds available. This route into the Hospital was made somewhat easier in 1809, when mandatory burial and clothing deposits, for poor patients in this category were abolished. They might also be admitted as paying patients, under the sponsorship of an agency such as the Philadelphia Almshouse, or as paying or poor patients, under the sponsorship of the Guardians of the Poor for Philadelphia County. A third way was to be sponsored by a private patron who might be an employer, or simply an acquaintance with a charitable bent.

Patients with physical afflictions were accommodated in crowded, open wards of up to twenty-five beds, without the benefit of a curtain for privacy. With the availability of increased varieties of fresh produce and meat—much of which continued to be raised by the Hospital— patients' diets were more varied than in the eighteenth century.[42] Although the patients at Eighth and Pine were more carefully screened than those at some other charitable institutions, there continued to be some problems with unruly behavior. Indeed, in 1816, an adult male patient was charged with the attempted rape of an eight year old female patient.[43]

Medical Treatment

Treatment of somatic illnesses varied according to the prescribing physician, but bleeding was universally prescribed, with doctors Rush and Physick being joined by Physick's nephew, Dr. John Syng Dorsey, as the leading exponents of this practice. Although the importance of cleanliness was not yet universally recognized, the Hospital continued to employ a washerwoman. Nevertheless, the problems with puerperal fever may have been, in part, attributable to the lack of cleanliness in the lying-in department.

Medicine was going through an awkward period in which the old "systems" of the eighteenth century were being discarded, but new theories, based on the belief that microorganisms caused disease, were still far in the future. The one field of medicine that did seem to make considerable strides during the first half of the nineteenth century was surgery. Although the introduction of anesthesia would be a post 1841 development, the number of operations at Eighth and Pine showed a considerable increase over the previous century. Prior to 1800, there were only twelve lithotomies, while from 1800 to 1841, sixty-two were performed. Although exact figures on the total number of surgical operations during the first four decades of the nineteenth century are not available, the development of new techniques by the Hospital's surgeons encouraged an increase in operations. But the danger of infection continued to deter deep incisions into the thoracic and stomach cavities.

For the patient it must have been a terrifying experience to be brought into the Hospital's operating ampitheatre which might be filled, if the upcoming surgery was of a particularly interesting nature, with almost 300 onlookers. Because of the excruciating pain and related physiological problems, the mark of a good surgeon continued to be his quickness with the knife. To the suffering patient the substitutes for anesthesia (laudanum, whiskey etc.) and the promise of quickness, did little to ease the apprehension as the patient looked around the sky-lighted amphitheatre. The skylight did not, however, give enough illumination for minute surgical work and Doctor Physick and other surgeons had to perform eye operations in another room.[44]

Standard procedure dictated that the patient be tied down to the operating table, and then held from moving by strong-armed attendants, although in at least one case the attendants weren't needed. A small boy, about to be cut for the stone, promised everyone that he would remain perfectly still if he could smoke a cigar during the operation. "He bore the cutting with impressive tranquility."[45]

The Insane

The insane patients were housed in individual cells in the west wing, with the Hospital doing its best to segregate males from females, and the extremely unruly from the rest. The wealthier insane—these included Rush's son; painter Charles Wilson Peale's daughter; the sister of Louis McLane, Andrew Jackson's Secretary of State; the brother of Henry Knox, Washington's first Secretary of War; and Stephen Girard's wife—were sometimes attended by a private servant, given separate quarters, and were otherwise segregated from the other patients. This special treatment contrasted with eighteenth century practices, but is understandable in view of the extraordinarily high fee charged these patients—in some cases it amounted to $10.00 per week—and the fact that service to patients of this type served to advertise the Hospital in certain important quarters.

Treatment of insane patients tended to move away from Benjamin Rush's regimen of bleeding, purging and sweating, and by 1840, this regimen was almost totally abandoned at Eighth and Pine. In its place, the new moral treatment, so popular with European reformers, was adopted. Moral treatment, with its emphasis on kindness and lack of restraints, led to the Hospital giving employment to the insane, and encouraging them to take part in games and exercises, in fenced in yards set aside for that purpose. Diverting the attention of the insane from their problems was felt essential, and attendants were instructed to read to them and to procure books for those who could read.

Violently insane patients continued to be a problem, ripping up their beds, destroying furniture, attacking attendants and physicians, and even committing suicide. Because it was felt that the insane could be most easily cured if they were admitted and treated immediately after the onslaught of their affliction, the Hospital urged the public to think of the Hospital as an institution of first rather than last resort. Nevertheless, the continued indiscriminate admission of visitors to the insane department caused one young patient, tired of being a public spectacle, to discharge a musketball "through his head," and made many prospective patients and their families, hesitant about seeking an early solution to their problem at Eighth and Pine. Benjamin Rush was particularly cognizant of this problem and constantly urged the Board to more carefully screen visitors, but the problem continued to occupy the attention of the Board long after Rush's death.[46]

A Look at the Record

Despite less than ideal physical accommodations, the Hospital continued to claim good results in treating its patients. The mortality rate for resident patients from 1801 to 1841, ran in the neighborhood of 9 percent, which was lower than the eighteenth century figure but similar to the mortality rate in the New York Hospital for the same period.[47]

Although its performance was satisfactory when measured by its mortality rate, the Pennsylvania Hospital did not exercise leadership in medical research, an area that was becoming an increasingly important hospital function. While a few of the Hospital's medical staff did introduce advances in their specialties, a certain medical conservatism was setting in at Eighth and Pine. Indicative of this pervading suspicion of change, was the Hospital's feet dragging on the development of a lying-in department, and the building of a separate asylum for the insane, as well as lying-in physician Charles Meigs' rejection of the progressive view that puerperal fever was infectious.

It is not surprising then, that when the new research-oriented ideas from Paris crossed the Atlantic in the early nineteenth century, they were greeted with less enthusiasm at Eighth and Pine, than at some other American hospitals. As a result, by the 1820's and 1830's, the Pennsylvania Hospital was taking a back seat to the Massachusetts General and the Philadelphia General (Blockley) in the area of medical research. Thus by 1841, Anglo-America's first hospital was no longer the nation's largest, nor its leader, in pioneering new methods of treatment, via research, for its patients.[48]

Chapter 8

Conclusion

Philanthropy has rarely been as disinterested as its benefactors would have us believe. In medieval times, the pervading interest in a heavenly reward, greatly influenced the purpose of philanthropy. Benefactors gave generously to charity, not so much because they were interested in alleviating misery and injustice, but rather because they wished to impress a merciful God of their fitness for a heavenly destination. The impact of philanthropic giving, therefore, was of little import to medieval benefactors. By contrast, modern philanthropy is infected with the secular spirit of the times and is, therefore, very much concerned with the impact of its beneficences on society, or at least on small segments thereto. To the modern benefactor, it is this world that really counts and his philanthropic giving is aimed at shaping this world, or at least part of it, to reflect his own assumptions as to what is best for society. In short, modern philanthropy is often just another way that the rich and the wellborn force their will on the humble and unfortunate.

The Pennsylvania Hospital grew out of this modern philanthropic tradition, with its emphasis on charity as a means of shaping society in a desired way. Using a stick and carrot technique, the Hospital tried to encourage a respect for the work ethic and for high moral standards among Pennsylvania's poor. Quite simply put, those poor who worked hard, and had good character references, were rewarded by admission as nonpaying patients, as long as they could meet the other admission criteria. However, those who were equally poor but not as deserving— that is, lacking in industriousness and morality—were turned away or had to find a sympathetic patron or another institution to pay for their stay at Eighth and Pine. Of course the admission of the insane was based on different criteria, but that was because so many diverse factors were involved in the decision to institutionalize Pennsylvania's "lunatics."

Because it patterned itself after the provincial voluntary hospitals of Great Britain, the Pennsylvania Hospital was not a new and unique institution in the Turnerian sense. Indeed, by the nineteenth century, a certain conservatism had crept into Thomas Bond's pioneer institution, causing the Hospital to be less adventuresome and more hidebound than most other contemporary American hospitals. Despite the fact that the number of patients and the size of the capital stock were constantly on

148

the increase, a hardening of the arteries was setting in at Eighth and Pine, and this disease of old age caused the Hospital to hold back, when it should have dared innovate, to ignore new ideas when it should have been eagerly examining them. Nevertheless, the opening of the new insane department west of the Schuylkill in 1841, marked a break with the business as usual attitudes that had characterized the recent past. The new physical expansion would stimulate new thinking about the future which, in turn, might even conjure up a renewal of the pioneering spirit, that characterized the Pennsylvania Hospital during much of the eighteenth century.

Appendix

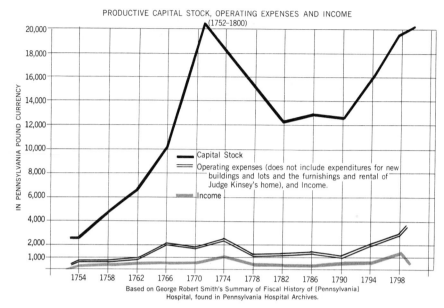

PRODUCTIVE CAPITAL STOCK, OPERATING EXPENSES AND INCOME
(1752–1800)

Capital Stock

Operating expenses (does not include expenditures for new buildings and lots and the furnishings and rental of Judge Kinsey's home), and Income.

Income

Based on George Robert Smith's Summary of Fiscal History of [Pennsylvania] Hospital, found in Pennsylvania Hospital Archives.

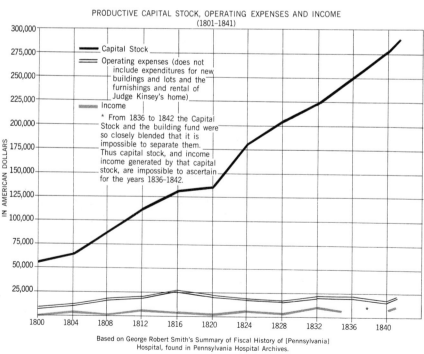

PRODUCTIVE CAPITAL STOCK, OPERATING EXPENSES AND INCOME
(1801–1841)

Capital Stock

Operating expenses (does not include expenditures for new buildings and lots and the furnishings and rental of Judge Kinsey's home)

Income

* From 1836 to 1842 the Capital Stock and the building fund were so closely blended that it is impossible to separate them. Thus capital stock, and income income generated by that capital stock, are impossible to ascertain for the years 1836–1842.

Based on George Robert Smith's Summary of Fiscal History of [Pennsylvania] Hospital, found in Pennsylvania Hospital Archives.

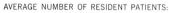

AVERAGE NUMBER OF RESIDENT PATIENTS:
(1752–1841)

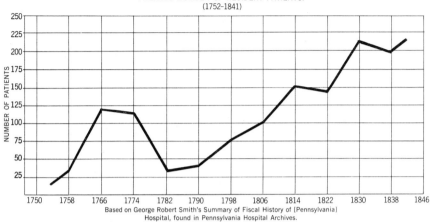

Based on George Robert Smith's Summary of Fiscal History of [Pennsylvania]
Hospital, found in Pennsylvania Hospital Archives.

AVERAGE NUMBER OF POOR AND PAYING PATIENTS IN RESIDENCE
(1752–1841)

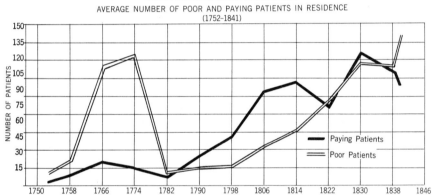

Based on Bd. of M.M., I–IX and Rough Minutes 1781–1801.

AVERAGE NUMBER OF PATIENTS IN RESIDENCE BROKEN DOWN INTO INSANE AND NON-INSANE
CATEGORIES (1753–1841)

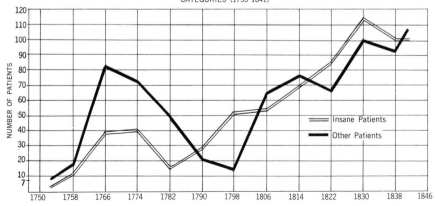

Based on Bd. of M.M. I–VII, Rough Minutes, 1753–1801, and Annual Reports,
1794–1841. Omitted in the plotting of all the graphs were all non-civilian patients.

Notes

Chapter 1

1. *Pennsylvania Gazette,* March 18, 1731; August 8, 1751.
2. Carl and Jessica Bridenbaugh, *Rebels and Gentlemen: Philadelphia in the Age of Franklin* (New York, 1962), 2–4. Bridenbaugh maintains that Philadelphia was the second largest city in the British Empire, but he probably ignored some of the Empire's non-English speaking cities such as those of India. Philadelphia became the largest city in the English colonies in North America by 1760, when she surpassed Boston's population. *Ibid.,* 5. More recent research on colonial Philadelphia's population disagrees with Bridenbaugh's figures but does point up Philadelphia's rapid growth during the colonial period. See, for example, Gary B. Nash and Bill G. Smith, "Population and Eighteenth Century Philadelphia," *Pa. Mag. of Hist. and Bio.,* July 1975, 362–368.
3. William C. Heffner, *History of Poor Relief Legislation in Pennsylvania* (Cleona, Pa., 1912), 67, 68, 73.
4. Bridenbaugh, *Rebels and Gentlemen,* 230.
5. Richard H. Shryock, *Medicine and Society in America, 1660–1860* (Ithaca, N.Y., 1962), 84; *Pennsylvania Archives,* 8th ser., IV, 3403; John Smith's Diaries, IX, August 30, October 9, 23, 1750, Library Company Collection, Historical Society of Pennsylvania. Board of Managers Minutes, Pennsylvania Hospital Archives, I, 23, 84. Hereafter Board of Managers Minutes will be referred to as Bd. of M.M. The papers of the Pennsylvania Hospital have been microfilmed and are available at the American Philosophical Society, Philadelphia. The Pennsylvania Hospital Archives are in the Pine Street building on Eighth and Pine, Philadelphia.
6. Elizabeth H. Thomson, "Thomas Bond, 1713–1784: First Professor of Clinical Medicine in the American Colonies," *Journal of Medical Education,* XXXIII, no. 9, 614–624; Sydney James, *A People Among Peoples, Quaker Benevolence in Eighteenth Century America* (Cambridge, Mass., 1963), 206. Theodore Thayer in *Israel Pemberton: King of the Quakers* (Philadelphia, 1943), n36, states "Dr. Phineas Bond had urged the founding of a hospital for sometime and was, no doubt, instrumental in awakening Quaker interest." I suspect that Mr. Thayer may have been misled into giving Phineas Bond the credit due his brother Thomas Bond, because of an error in *Guide to the Manuscript Collections, Historical Society of Pennsylvania* (Philadelphia, 1940), no. 64, which refers to Phineas Bond as a founder of the Pennsylvania Hospital.

    Thomas Bond was probably disowned by the Philadelphia Monthly Meeting for marrying out of unity. However, there is no extant record of the exact charge beyond "disunity with Friends." Thomson, 623.
7. Benjamin Franklin, *The Autobiography and Other Writings,* ed. L. Jesse Lemisch (New York, 1961), 133. In Franklin's *Some Account of the Pennsylvania Hospital,* ed. I. Bernard Cohen (Baltimore, 1954), 3, the date for the conception of the idea for the hospital is given as late 1750.
8. *Pennsylvania Archives,* 8th ser., IV, 3403; Thomas G. Morton and Frank Woodbury, *History of the Pennsylvania Hospital* (Philadelphia, 1897), 8; Leonard W. Labaree, ed., *The Papers of Benjamin Franklin,* V (New Haven, Conn., 1961), 285, 286.
9. *Pennsylvania Archives,* 8th ser., IV, 3407, 3412; Franklin, *The Autobiography and Other Writings,* 133, 134. Franklin's proposal that the government match funds raised by private contributions to support a hospital was not new. In London in 1544, funds for St. Bartholomew's Hospital were raised in this manner.
10. Franklin, *The Autobiography and Other Writings,* ed. Lemisch, 134, 135.

11. *Colonial Records,* 1st ser., V, 526; *Pennsylvania Archives,* 8th ser., IV, 3431, 3432.

12. Bd. of M.M., I, 1; Frederick Tolles, *Meeting House and Counting House: The Quaker Merchants of Colonial Philadelphia, 1682–1763* (New York, 1963), 131, n60, gives a list of Quaker grandees prior to the American Revolution. Tolles' list can be supplemented by use of proprietary tax figures for 1769 found in *Pennsylvania Archives,* 3rd ser., XIV.

13. Franklin, *Some Account of the Pennsylvania Hospital,* ed. Cohen, 5–7. The Hospital charter is also printed in full in Morton and Woodbury, *History of the Pennsylvania Hospital,* 9–11. Bd. of M.M., I, 1, 2.

14. Although there were two proprietors during the 1750's (Thomas Penn and his brother Richard Penn), in 1746 Thomas Penn acquired a three-fourths interest in the colony and, henceforth, made the vital decisions concerning Pennsylvania. Although the Managers sometimes spoke of proprietors rather than proprietor, this was merely a matter of correct form.

15. Penn Manuscripts, Official Correspondence, V, 1967, Historical Society of Pennsylvania; Bd. of M.M., I, 34, 35, 3, 36, 37.

16. Franklin, *Some Account of the Pennsylvania Hospital,* ed. Cohen, 5–7.

17. Bd. of M.M., I, 7, 13, 30, 47. For an idea of Israel Pemberton's wealth see *Pennsylvania Archives,* 3rd ser., XIV, 183.

18. Bd. of M.M., I, 8, 13, 14. Edwin Bronner, "The Disgrace of John Kinsey, Quaker Politician, 1739–1750, "*Pennsylvania Magazine of History and Biography,* LXXV (1951), 403–414. This method of starting a hospital in a private home certainly had a precedent. Without many exceptions, British voluntary hospitals began this way.

19. Bd. of M.M., I, 14, 16, 23.

20. Franklin, *Some Account of the Pennsylvania Hospital,* ed. Cohen, 5; Bd. of M.M., I, 15. After a staff of six attending physicians was appointed in May of 1752, the Hospital no longer appointed a consulting staff.

21. Bd. of M.M., I, 19. For a printed copy of the regulations see Morton and Woodbury, *History of the Pennsylvania Hospital,* 29–32.

22. Bd. of M.M., I, 38, 40; Steward's Cash Book, Jan. 1, 1772, Feb. 22, 1772, March 28, 1772.

23. W. H. McMenemey, "The Hospital Movement of the Eighteenth Century and Its Development," *The Evolution of Hospitals in Britain,* ed. F. N. L. Poynter (London, 1964), 57.

24. Alured Clarke, *A Collection of Papers Relating to the County Hospital for Sick and Lame at Winchester* (London, 1737), x; *Gentleman's Magazine,* XI (London, 1741), 474; XII (London, 1742), 152; XIII (London, 1743), 640; XIV (London, 1744), 52; *An Account of the Public Hospital for the Diseased Poor in the County of York* (York, 1743), 3.

25. Franklin, *Some Account of the Pennsylvania Hospital,* ed. Cohen, 4.

26. *Pennsylvania Gazette* (Philadelphia), Aug. 8, 1751; Aug. 15, 1751.

27. *Gentleman's Magazine,* VI (London, 1736), 618; VII (London, 1737), 636; IX (London, 1739), 408; XI (London, 1741), 474, 497, 652; XII (London, 1742), 152; XIII (London, 1743), 640; XIV (London, 1744), 52; XVIII (London, 1748, 198; Verner W. Crane, *Benjamin Franklin and a Rising People* (Boston, 1954), 25.

28. Alured Clarke, *A Collection of Papers Relating to the County Hospital for Sick and Lame at Winchester;* W. H. McMenemey, "The Hospital Movement of the Eighteenth Century and Its Development," *The Evolution of Hospitals in Great Britain,* ed. Poynter, 53.

29. Occasional references indicate that a systematic effort by the Pennsylvania Hospital to collect material on contemporary British hospitals was underway at an early date. Bd. of M.M., I, 147; James Pemberton to William Logan, Feb. 5, 1761, Pemberton Copy Book, 1740–1780, 199, Historical Society of Pennsylvania.

30. *A Letter From a Gentleman in Town to His Friend in the Country Relating to the Royal Infirmary of Edinburgh* (Edinburgh, 1749), 1.

31. James Thacher, *American Medical Biography* (Boston, 1828), 179. Carl and Jessica Bridenbaugh in *Rebels and Gentleman*, 244, maintain that Thomas Bond visited England in 1748, returning to Philadelphia in the same year full of such enthusiasm for the English hospital movement that he immediately proposed establishment of a hospital in Philadelphia. Actually, Thomas Bond left Philadelphia in 1748, but his destination was Barbadoes, his purpose to improve his health. John Ross to Cadwalader Evans, Nov. 13, 1748, *Pennsylvania Magazine of History and Biography*, XIII (1889), 381–382. The fact that Thomas Bond did not travel to England in 1748, was called to my attention by Elizabeth Thomson of the Yale University School of Medicine.

32. *Pennsylvania Gazette* (Philadelphia), Aug. 8, 1751; A. Logan Turner, *The Story of a Great Hospital, The Royal Infirmary of Edinburgh* (London, 1937), 84.

33. John Bellers, *An Essay Towards the Improvement of Physick in Twelve Proposals* (London, 1714), passim; David Owen, *English Philanthropy, 1660–1960* (Cambridge, Mass., 1964), 40; *Pennsylvania Gazette*, Aug. 8, 1751.

34. Alured Clarke, *A Proposal For Erecting a Public Hospital* (Winchester, 1736), 5; *Gentleman's Magazine*, IX (London, 1741), 475; XIII (London, 1743), 640; Richard Grey, *A Sermon for the Sick and Lame at Northampton County Infirmary* (Northampton, 1744), 16; *Pennsylvania Gazette*, Aug. 15, 1751.

35. *Gentleman's Magazine*, XIII (London, 1743), 640; Franklin, *Some Account of the Pennsylvania Hospital*, ed. Cohen, 3.

36. The incorporation of the Overseers of the Poor was aimed at keeping down Philadelphia's poor rates by allowing the Overseers to accept private contributions, thus enabling private philanthropy to shoulder some of the burden of public charity. William Clinton Heffner, *History of Poor Relief Legislation in Pennsylvania, 1682–1913* (Cleona, Pa., 1903), 73, 74.

37. Alured Clarke, *A Sermon Preached in the Cathedral Church of Winchester . . . 1736* (London, 1737), 8; Grey, *A Sermon for the Sick and Lame at Northampton County Infirmary*, 20, 21.

38. Bd. of M.M., I, 39.

39. Dorothy Marshall, *The English Poor in the Eighteenth Century* (London, 1926), 13, 14, 22, 23; Alured Clarke, *A Collection of Papers Relating to the County Hospital for Sick and Lame at Winchester*, iv, xiv; Clarke, *A Proposal for Erecting a Public Hospital*, 1.

40. Albert Henry Smyth, ed., *The Writings of Benjamin Franklin*, V (New York, 1907), 123.

41. Up until mid-century, Quakers in Pennsylvania were not much different in their charitable benevolence than other colonial sectarian groups. Generally, Quaker philanthropy was aimed at helping fellow Quakers. The one Philadelphia institution that the Quakers did establish prior to 1751 in the field of poor relief was an almshouse exclusively for the use of Quaker unfortunates. For a discussion of the change in Quaker attitudes towards institutional charity see Sydney James, *A People Among Peoples: Quaker Benevolence in Eighteenth Century America* (Cambridge, Mass., 1963).

42. A. G. R. Smith, *The Government of Elizabethan England* (New York, 1967), 80; Marcus W. Jernigan, *Laboring and Dependent Classes in Colonial America, 1607–1783* (Chicago, 1931), 191; Samuel Mencher, *Poor Law to Poverty Program* (Pittsburgh, 1967), 22, 23.

43. Labaree ed., *The Papers of Benjamin Franklin*, IV, 482. As might be expected, a workhouse was established in Philadelphia in 1767 to promote industry and frugality among the poor. Bridenbaugh, *Rebels and Gentlemen; Philadelphia in the Age of Franklin*, 232.

44. Grey, *A Sermon for the Sick and Lame at Northampton County Infirmary*, 15; Thomas Holme, *A Sermon . . .* (Northampton, 1745), 27; John, Lord Bishop of Peterborough, *A Sermon . . .* (Northampton, 1748), 18; John Nixon, *A Sermon . . .* (Northampton, 1749), 14.

45. Clarke, *A Proposal for Erecting a Public Hospital*, 7, 4; Grey, *A Sermon for the Sick and Lame at Northampton County Infirmary*, 13.

46. *Gentleman's Magazine*, XI (London, 1741), 476; Holm, *A Sermon . . .*, 27; Subscription Book, Bristol Royal Infirmary Archives, Bristol, England, 1; *An Account of the Public Hospital for the Diseased Poor in the County of York* (York, 1743), 2; Henry Layng, *A Sermon . . .* (Northampton, 1749), 14; Isaac, Lord Bishop . . ., *The Duty and Advantages of Encouraging Public Infirmaries: A Sermon . . .* (London, 1743), passim.

47. *An Account of the Rise and Establishmnt of the Infirmary, Or Hospital for the Sick-poor, Erected at Edinburgh* (Edinburgh, 1730), 11.

48. Sick-poor applicants to most eighteenth century British hospitals had to be suffering from a "curable," noncontagious malady before they could be admitted. The precedent for refusing incurables to British hospitals had been established in the seventeenth century. Contagious diseases were barred from the Pennsylvania Hospital, but some incurable insane patients were admitted. Bd. of M.M., I, 38.

49. Jackson Turner Main, *The Social Structure of Revolutionary America* (Princeton, 1965), 157; John K. Alexander, "The City of Brotherly Fear," *Cities in American History*, eds. K. Jackson and S. Schultz (New York, 1972), 81. For the view that most colonists did not make this distinction see Main, 198. For papers of some of the most important founders of the Pennsylvania Hospital see Coates-Reynell Papers, Pemberton Papers and John Smith's Diaries, in the Historical Society of Pennsylvania. Franklin became even less sympathetic towards the poor in his later years. See Howell V. Williams, "Benjamin Franklin and the Poor Laws," *Social Science Review*, XVIII (1944), 77-91.

50. Franklin, "The Act to Encourage the Establishing of an Hospital for the Relief of the Sick Poor of This Province, and for the Reception and Cure of Lunatics," *Some Account of the Pennsylvania Hospital*, ed. Cohen, 5; Franklin, *The Autobiography and Other Writings*, ed. Lemisch, 134. Although, as noted in n49, Franklin became increasing critical of the poor he, nevertheless, continued to hold the Pennsylvania Hospital in high esteem. *Ibid.*, 134, 135.

51. Crane, *Benjamin Franklin and a Rising People* (Boston, 1954), 30; Judy M. DiStefano, A Concept of the Family in Colonial America: The Pembertons of Philadelphia (Ph.D. dissertation, Ohio State University, 1970), 275, 278, passim; Carl L. Romanek, John Reynell, Quaker Merchant of Philadelphia (Ph.D. dissertation, Pennsylvania State University, 1969), passim.

52. Bd. of M.M., I, 38, 39.

53. Entrees for April 3, June 16, 1794, Book of Daily Occurrency, House of Employment and Almshouse of Philadelphia, March 25, 1794–Sept. 28, 1795, on microfilm courtesy of Dale Fields, Historical Society of Delaware, Wilmington, Del.; Bd. of M.M., I-VII; Rough Minutes, 1753–1801, Pennsylvania Hospital Archives. This is not to say that only those with unimpeachable character were allowed into Anglo-America's first hospital. Certainly, if there were empty beds and enough money available to support those beds, less desirable types were also admitted.

54. *Gentleman's Magazine*, XI (London, 1741), 476, 477.

55. Bd. of M.M., I, 39.

56. *The History and Statutes of the Royal Infirmary of Edinburgh* (Edinburgh, 1778), 27; Susan Fairclough, The Royal Infirmary of Edinburgh, 1770–1775, 8 (unpublished paper), Archives of Royal Infirmary of Edinburgh.

57. Bd. of M.M., I, 39.

58. *Ibid.*, 83–87.

Chapter 2

1. James Hamilton to Thomas Penn, July 5, 1751, Penn Manuscripts, Official Correspondence, V, 167, Historical Society of Pennsylvania.

2. Tolles, *Meeting House and Counting House: The Quaker Merchants of Colonial Philadelphia, 1682–1763*, 49, 228, 231–233; Bd. of M.M., I-IV, passim; William

Wade Hinshaw, *Encyclopedia of American Quaker Genealogy* (Ann Arbor, Mich., 1938), II, passim; and citings from a number of different monographs dealing with the period. In a few cases I may have counted as Quakers some who were no longer in good standing with their Meeting, but I also, no doubt, overlooked a few Managers who should have been classified as Quakers. The cited statistics, therefore, may not give as exact a picture as I would like, but they are, in an approximate sense, correct.

3. Specific examples of Quaker participation in the British voluntary hospital movement can be found in the hospitals at Bath, Exeter, Bristol and London.

4. James, *A People Among Peoples*, 193–207.

5. William S. Hanna, *Benjamin Franklin and Pennsylvania Politics* (Stanford, Cal., 1964), 52.

6. Thomas Penn's Letterbook, III, 139, 87, Historical Society of Pennsylvania.

7. John F. Watson, Annals of Philadelphia, Supplement Annal, 31, 32, Historical Society of Pennsylvania; Morton and Woodbury, *History of the Pennsylvania Hospital*, 17–20; Bd. of M.M., I, 27, 48–52.

8. Morton and Woodbury, *History of the Pennsylvania Hospital*, 21; Bd. of M.M., I, 51–53.

9. Bd. of M.M., I, 51–53; Morton and Woodbury, *History of the Pennsylvania Hospital*, 20, 21. Thomas Penn, when informed of the Board's apprehension, told intermediaries Hyam and Bevan that any buildings erected on the plot granted by the Proprietors would revert to the Board of Managers. When asked by Bevan and Hyam to put this assurance in writing, however, Thomas Penn refused. Bd. of M.M., I, 88.

10. Thayer, *Israel Pemberton: King of the Quakers*, 60, 61; Hanna, *Benjamin Franklin and Pennsylvania Politics*, 210, n26; Manuscript Letters from Thomas Penn to Richard Peters and Others, 1752–1772, Peters' Papers, 6, Historical Society of Pennsylvania. Back in 1739 Israel Pemberton, Jr., had been arrested for criticizing Thomas Penn but the case was eventually dropped. See Edward M. Bailey in *D.A.B.* s.v. Pemberton, Israel., 412.

11. Thayer, *Israel Pemberton*, 134. Israel Pemberton's volatile nature reveals itself in his correspondence found in the Pemberton Papers and Etting Collection, passim, Historical Society of Pennsylvania. For an idea of Pemberton's social circle see John Smith's Diaries, Library Company Collection, Historical Society of Pennsylvania. For a view of the two Quaker factions see James Hutson, "Benjamin Franklin and Pennsylvania Politics, 1751–1755; A Reappraisal," *Pennsylvania Magazine of History and Biography*, XCIII (1969), 312, 313.

12. Thomas Penn's Letter Book, III, 168, Historical Society of Pennsylvania; Manuscript Letters from Thomas Penn to Richard Peters and Others, 1752–1772, Peter's Papers, 24, Historical Society of Pennsylvania; *Pennsylvania Archives*, 8th ser., IV, 3569; Morton and Woodbury, *History of the Pennsylvania Hospital*, 23. Hanna in *Benjamin Franklin and Pennsylvania Politics*, 17, supports the view that Thomas Penn was deeply concerned with the well-being of Pennsylvania.

13. Bd. of M.M., I, 88; Watson, Annals of Philadelphia, Supplement Annal, 32, Historical Society of Pennsylvania.

14. Thomas Penn's Letter Book, VII, 126, Historical Society of Pennsylvania; Bd. of M.M., II, 405. William Logan, a member of the Provincial Council and friend of the Penns, may have been the key person in establishing harmony between the Hospital and the Proprietor because Logan was also cousin to Israel Pemberton. Logan later became a Hospital Manager. John W. Jordan, ed., *Colonial Families of Philadelphia* (New York, 1911), I, 30, 31. After the American Revolution the Penn family—albeit the American branch—continued the generous though tardy example of the Proprietor. In 1788, John Penn, nephew of Thomas Penn, and John Penn, Jr., contributed between them almost $350 to the Hospital. Bd. of M.M., VI, 208; Morton and Woodbury, *History of the Pennsylvania Hospital*, 393.

15. According to James Hutson in "Benjamin Franklin and Pennsylvania Politics, 1751–1755: A Reappraisal," *Pennsylvania Magazine of History and Biography,* July, 1969, 317, 318, Franklin kept in check his Whiggish leanings and, therefore did not take an anti-proprietary stance during the early 1750's in order to promote two of his most ambitious philanthropic undertakings: The Academy and the Pennsylvania Hospital. But once both institutions were on their feet, Franklin's Whiggish political convictions no longer had to be restrained. By contrast, while Franklin became a staunch foe of proprietary government, Israel Pemberton began a reappraisal of proprietary government. By the early 1760's, with the French and Indian war coming to an end, Pemberton became a lukewarm supporter of proprietary government. Thayer, *Israel Pemberton,* 202, 203.

16. Bd. of M.M., I, 139, 143, 146. Morton and Woodbury, *History of the Pennsylvania Hospital,* 36, maintain that the purchase price was £100. The Free Society of Traders had originally received a grant of 199 acres in Philadelphia from William Penn. The tract of land ran between Pine and Spruce Streets from the Delaware to the Schuylkill.

17. Bd. of M.M., I, 146, 147, 151; Tolles, *Meeting House and Counting House,* 94; Jordan, *Colonial Families in Philadelphia,* I, 319. Other builders among the contributors included Quakers Robert Smith and Samuel Powell. Robert Smith and Samuel Rhoads later worked together in planning and constructing the Philadelphia Bettering House (Almshouse) in 1766 and 1767. Bridenbaugh, *Rebels and Gentlemen,* 199–202.

18. Engraving is in the Archives of the Pennsylvania Hospital.

19. This is an assumption based on the fact that Rhoads was the finer architect and that Fox would act out of deference to his colleague's wishes. Another reason for suspecting Rhoads as the primary initiator of the overall plan is the similarity between the Hospital plan and the "bettering House" which Rhoads probably had a hand in designing. See n17. Once planning for the eastern wing commenced it was quite obvious that Rhoads was in command.

20. The term "unornamental functionalism" is used by Bridenbaugh to describe Rhoads' architectural style. Bridenbaugh, *Rebels and Gentlemen,* 200.

21. William Adam, *Vitruvius Scoticus* (Edinburgh, 1750), plates 149, 150; John D. Comrie, *History of Scottish Medicine to 1860* (London, 1927), 125, 127; Richard M. Candee, Philadelphia Hospital Design, 1754–1844, (unpublished course paper, University of Pennsylvania), 3. The London Hospital, another logical source of inspiration, seemed so different from the Pennsylvania Hospital in its interior design that Rhoads was probably little influenced by its example. A. E. Clarke-Kennedy, *The London,* 122.

22. Turner, *The Story of a Great Hospital, The Royal Infirmary of Edinburgh, 1729–1939,* 79, 80, 83. The second oldest hospital in the thirteen colonies, the New York, founded in 1773, was also based on the architectural plan of the Edinburgh Infirmary. Patrick M'Robert, *A Tour Through Part of the North Provinces of America, 1774–1775,* ed., Carl Bridenbaugh (Philadelphia, 1935), 3.

23. Bridenbaugh, *Rebels and Gentlemen,* 200.

24. Bd. of M.M., I, 152, 153. Samuel Rhoads' elevation is not extant.

25. One John Parrish presented himself as mason and bricklayer, and offered his services to the Managers in 1755. Evidently Parrish got the message concerning subscribers' privileges because he contributed £10 by the end of 1756. Bd. of M.M., I, 153; Morton and Woodbury, *History of the Pennsylvania Hospital,* 392.

26. The cornerstone reads "In the year of Christ, MDCCLV George the Second Happily Reigning (For he sought the happiness of his people) Philadelphia flourishing (for its inhabitants were public spirited) This building by the Bounty of the Government And of Many private persons was piously founded For relief of the Sick and Miserable; May the God of Mercies Bless the Undertaking." Morton and Woodbury, *History of the Pennsylvania Hospital,* 40; Bd. of M.M., I, 155, 191, 224.

27. *Ibid.*

28. The print of the Hospital's eastern wing and its bucolic setting is printed in

John Welsh Croskey, *History of Blockley* (Philadelphia, 1929), 18. The print is incorrectly labeled the Philadelphia Almshouse but a glance at a second print published, in Morton and Woodbury, *The History of the Pennsylvania Hospital,* 321, proves that the Croskey print was actually the eastern wing of the Pennsylvania Hospital as it appeared about 1768. This is not the first time that Croskey's book confuses the Almshouse with the Pennsylvania Hospital. In his introduction (p. 14) Croskey quotes from Manasseh Cutler in describing the early almshouse when Cutler was really describing the Pennsylvania Hospital.

29. Andrew Burnaby, *Burnaby's Travels Through North America, 1759, 1760,* ed., Rufus Rockwell Wilson (New York, 1904), 89; Edward B. Krumbhaar, "The Pennsylvania Hospital," ed., Luther P. Eisenhart, *Historic Philadelphia, from the Founding until the Early Nineteenth Century* (Philadelphia, 1953), 239.

30. Bd. of M.M., II, 199, 200; John Adams, *The Adams Papers: Diary and Autobiography,* ed., L. H. Butterfield (New York, 1964), II, 116. For other details of both the overall plan and the design of the east wing see Morton and Woodbury, *History of the Pennsylvania Hospital,* 37, 38.

31. Bd. of M.M., II, 200, 83, 112, 178.

32. *Ibid.,* 65, 409. Morton and Woodbury in *The History of The Pennsylvania Hospital,* 37, maintain that in the building of the Hospital "scarcely a tradesman was patronized, or even a workman employed, without his first pledging a donation or discount, or inducing him to become a contributor." I can find no record that the above represented official policy but a few small pieces of information—see for example n25—point to the possibility of this approach being used in many cases. Even Gilchrist and McCauley, the two offending craftsmen spoken of above, contributed together £6.66. Morton and Woodbury, *History of the Pennsylvania Hospital,* 372.

33. Thomas Penn to Richard Peters, September 28, 1751, Watson, Annals of Philadelphia, Supplement Annal, 31, 32, Historical Society of Pennsylvania.

34. Bd. of M.M., I, 129, III, 368, 231; Franklin, *Some Account of the Pennsylvania Hospital,* ed. Cohen, 39, 40. To figure the exact number of Contributors at any one time is impossible because, although names of the Contributors were recorded, their death dates were not. The 1754 figure is an approximation made possible by the relative youth of the Hospital which gave the Contributors little chance to die.

35. For an example of voter apathy in national elections for the same reason see Richard McCormick, *The Second American Party System: Party Formation in the Jackson Era* (Chapel Hill, N.C., 1966), 16.

36. Examples that come immediately to mind were Anglicans Evan Morgan and Jacob Duché. Hanna, *Benjamin Franklin and Pennsylvania Politics,* 104.

37. Thomas Penn to Richard Peters, September 28, 1751, Watson, Annals of Philadelphia, Supplement Annal, 31, 32, Historical Society of Pennsylvania; Bd. of M.M., I, 43. Richard Peters was very much involved in the Philadelphia Academy, being elected president of the Academy's Board of Trustees in 1756. For details on Richard Peter's two scandalous marriages in England as well as his subsequent rise to favor in Pennsylvania, see Hubertis Cummings, *Richard Peters* (Philadelphia, 1944).

38. Allen's initial contribution was £150 plus another £12 per year for life. By his death in 1780, William Allen had contributed $1,269.33 to the Hospital. Franklin, *Some Account of the Pennsylvania Hospital,* ed. Cohen, 39; Morton and Woodbury, *History of the Pennsylvania Hospital,* 377. Allen could exercise some influence over Hospital activities because, according to the Hospital charter, the laws and regulations of the Hospital were subject to the approval of the Chief Justice of Pennsylvania. Franklin, *Some Account of the Pennsylvania Hospital,* ed. Cohen, 6; Thayer, *Israel Pemberton,* 119.

39. *Ibid.,* 204, 205. James Pemberton to John Fothergill, December 18, 1765, Pemberton Copy Book, 1740–1780, Pemberton Papers, 253, Historical Society of Pennsylvania.

40. After atempting to quantify the occupations of a number of Managers, I found

it an impossible task. The extent of their wealth, however, is indicated in the Proprietary Tax Roll of 1769 found in *Pennsylvania Archives*, ser. 3, XIV.

41. Charles Lawrence, *History of the Philadelphia Almshouses and Hospitals* (Philadelphia, 1905), 22; Pemberton Copy Book, 1740–1780, Pemberton Papers, 197, Historical Society of Pennsylvania.

42. Tolles, *Meeting House and Counting House*, 229; Hanna, *Benjamin Franklin and Pennsylvania Politics*, 84. Franklin and Thomas Bond were exceptions to this generalization as these two non-Quakers helped found and continued to work for the success of the Academy.

43. Bd. of M.M., I, 179, 190.

44. *Pennsylvania Gazette*, Feb. 28, 1771.

45. Bd. of M.M., III, 192. See Bd. of M.M., I, 155, for examples of the Hospital's use of the *Gazette*.

46. Bd. of M.M., I, 218, 220, 225, 228. William S. Hanna, in *Benjamin Franklin and Pennsylvania Politics*, 116, places Franklin's departure from Philadelphia in February of 1757 but the wording of a resolution at a Managers' meeting on March 28, 1757, indicates that Franklin had not yet left. In Labaree, ed., *Papers of Benjamin Franklin*, VII, xxvi, the departure date from Philadelphia is given as April 8, 1757. Franklin was going to England as the agent of the Pennsylvania Assembly.

47. Franklin died in 1790 and left the Hospital all the unpaid debts owed him that the Hospital could collect. The Board met with the contributors and it was decided that because of the difficulty in recovering debts as old as those owed Franklin, the legacy should not be accepted. In 1792 the executors of the Franklin estate did present the Hospital "a curious bedstead." Bd. of M.M., VI, 314, 409. Franklin's activities in England on behalf of the Hospital are difficult to assess. Labaree, ed., *Papers of Benjamin Franklin* (New Haven, 1966), IX, 280, n.

48. Thayer, *Israel Pemberton*, 33.

49. Bd. of M.M., II, 141, 170, 240; Thayer, *Israel Pemberton*, 195n. Pemberton's objections to Weed were not spelled out in the Managers' Minutes.

50. Bd. of M.M., II, 141, 170.

51. Henry Biddle, "Colonial Mayors of Philadelphia; Samuel Rhoads," *Pennsylvania Magazine of History and Biography*, XIX, 68.

52. Since John Reynell served as Treasurer the first year of the Hospital's existence he had an excellent overview of the Hospital's fiscal and managerial problems.

53. Not to be confused with his cousin of the same name who became an active patriot during the American Revolution, serving as President of the Supreme Executive Council of Pennsylvania until his death in 1778. See James H. Peeling in *D.A.B.* s.v. "Wharton, Thomas."

54. Ernst Troeltsch, *The Social Teachings of the Christian Church*, trans. Olive Wyon (New York, 1931), II, 783. Marquis de Chastellux, *Travels in North America*, ed., Howard R. Rich (Chapel Hill, N.C., 1963), I, 130.

55. Labaree, ed., *Papers of Benjamin Franklin*, X, 82.

56. Pemberton Copy Book, 1740–1780, Pemberton Papers, 197, Historical Society of Pennsylvania; Thayer, *Israel Pemberton*, 205, 206, 227; Bd. of M.M., I–IV.

57. Charles Sydnor, *American Revolutionaries in the Making* (New York, 1962), 16.

58. The most recent reprinting of Franklin's *Some Account of the Pennsylvania Hospital* is the already cited ed., Cohen (Baltimore, 1954).

59. *Ibid.*, ix, x.

60. Bd. of M.M., I, 132, 135, 136.

61. *Ibid.*, 136, 126, 163, 164.

62. *Ibid.*, 58. Figures used to arrive at this total can be found in the Index to Bd. of M.M., I–IV under "Charity Boxes."

63. Bd. of M.M., I, 126, 163, 164; II, 77, 38, 39.

64. *Ibid.*, II, 82; *Pennsylvania Archives*, ser. 8, IV, 3553, VI, 4886. There were a

few friends of the Hospital in the Assembly in 1759. They included Daniel Roberdeau, Joseph Fox, and Speaker Isaac Norris.

65. *Pennsylvania Archives*, ser. 8, VI, 4906.

66. *Ibid.*, 4956, 5259; Bd. of M.M., II, 302. By the beginning of 1758, the cost of the building had almost reached the £3,000 estimate and there was much yet to be done. Bd. of M.M., II, 26. In 1759 the Assembly did grant the Hospital one-half of the penalties prescribed by "An Act to prevent the exportation of bad or unmerchantable staves, headings, boards and timbers." The Hospital's share under this act amounted to $215.00 or about £81 prior to the American Revolution. The Hospital was also granted three fourths of the fines levied by the Inspector of flour, which aggregated, prior to the Revolution, to $630 or approximately £236. *Pennsylvania Archives*, ser. 8, VI, 4990; Morton and Woodbury, *History of the Pennsylvania Hospital*, 248.

67. Bd. of M.M., II, 391, 392; Morton and Woodbury, *History of the Pennsylvania Hospital*, 248, 249.

68. Bd. of M.M., II, 351, 352, 203, 269. Printed copies of *Some Account of the Pennsylvania Hospital, 1754 to 1761*, can be found in he Archives of the Pennsylvania Hospital.

69. Bd. of M.M., I, 12, 32. Support from the German community for the Hospital is not surprising in view of the political alliance between the Quakers and Germans in colonial Pennsylvania.

70. Morton and Woodbury, *History of the Pennsylvania Hospital*, 49, 265-267; Bd. of M.M., II, 87, 159; III, 76, 77; IV, 163.

71. Bd. of M.M., II, 346, III, 190, 198; Morton and Woodbury, *History of the Pennsylvania Hospital*, 368; R. Hingston Fox, *Dr. John Fothergill and His Friends* (London, 1919), 370. Barclay donated £175 in 1762 while Fothergill, in addition to a gift of anatomical drawings and casts sent to the Hospital in 1762, donated £250 in 1765. These figures represent Pennsylvania currency as do all monetary figures mentioned in this paper, unless otherwise specified.

72. Bd. of M.M., III, 115–119, 151. That the Bevans were in affluent circumstances can't be doubted. Philadelphia physician Thomas Parke, while a student in England, visited Timothy Bevan's country home in 1771 and judged by the furniture of the house that Bevans was very rich. Whitfield Bell, Jr., "Thomas Parke's Student Life in England and Scotland, 1771–1773." *Pennsylvania Magazine of History and Biography*, LXXXV, 237. See also Desmond Chapman Huston and Ernest C. Cripps, *Through a City Archway: The Story of Allen and Hanburys, 1715–1954* (London, 1954), for more details on Sylvanus and Timothy Bevan. The £50 sterling, when turned into Pennsylvania currency amounted to upwards of £80. See Bd. of M.M., IV, 91.

73. Bd. of M.M., IV, 22, 72, 78, 267, 279, 372.

74. Fox, *Dr. John Fothergill and His Friends*, 373; Bd. of M.M., II, 197, 198.

75. Bd. of M.M., II, 435; III, 143; IV, 105, 109, 160, 199. £8,637 sterling was approximately £14,337 Pennsylvania currency. Bd. of M.M., IV, 204.

76. *Ibid.*, I, 13; II, 38; IV, 289, 349, 353. All annual financial reports up to 1775 were checked to verify this generalization. The financial reports appear in Bd. of M.M., I-IV.

77. *Ibid.*, II, 38; IV, 349, 353. Again, all annual financial reports up to 1775 were checked to verify this generalization. The financial reports appear in Bd. of M.M., I-IV.

78. Bd. of M.M., I-IV.

79. *Ibid.*, II, 38, 93, 94, 39; IV, 347–350, 353. A separate building fund paid for much of the cost of the early Hospital building program, but this fund ceased to exist in 1761. Bd. of M.M., II, 224, 225.

80. Morton and Woodbury, *History of the Pennsylvania Hospital*, 267, 262; Bd. of M.M., I, 66; III, 81; Frederick B. Tolles, *Quakers and the Atlantic Culture* (New York, 1960), 91-113.

81. Tolles, *Meeting House and Counting House*, 197; *Pennsylvania Gazette*, Decem-

27, 1759; Bd. of M.M., II, 141, 142. The Hospital received £47 from the play.

82. Scharf and Westcott, *History of Philadelphia*, I, 212.

83. Voltaire, *Candide*, ed., Alex Szogyi (New York, 1962), 204.

Chapter 3

1. Bd. of M.M., I, 40–41.

2. Whitfield Bell, Jr., *John Morgan, Continental Doctor* (Philadelphia, 1965), 118.

3. See for example Daniel J. Boorstin, *The Americans, The Colonial Experience* (New York, 1958), 213–219.

4. Those receiving their medical degrees from the University of Edinburgh were John Morgan, Samuel Preston Moore and Adam Kuhn.

5. Elizabeth Thomson, "Thomas Bond, 1713–84," *Journal of Medical Education*, XXXIII, no. 9 (1958), 622; Thacher, *American Medical Biography*, 212, 31, 265; Bridenbaugh, *Rebels and Gentlemen*, 273. Iliac Passion referred to the practice of giving patients quicksilver and drastic purgatives. Cadwalader recommended instead mild cathartics and the use of opiates. The title of Cadwalader's work on lead poisoning was *An Essay on the West India Dry Gripes, with the Method of Preventing and Curing That Cruel Distemper*. Dry gripes referred to the symptoms of lead poisoning which came from the leaden pipes used in distillation of Jamaica rum often used in making punch. George Norris, *The Early History of Medicine in Philadelphia* (Philadelphia, 1886), 23.

6. For the many activities of John Morgan see the biography by Whitfield Bell, Jr., mentioned above in n2.

7. Of the five physicians offering courses in the medical school, Thomas Bond was already a Hospital physician while John Morgan would be elected to the staff in 1773, Adam Kuhn in 1774, William Shippen, Jr., in 1778, and Benjamin Rush in 1783.

8. Bd. of M.M., I, 73; II, 117; IV, 252, 263, 317.

9. The Quakers were Lloyd Zachary, Samuel Preston Moore, Cadwalader Evans and Charles Moore. The former Quakers were the Bond brothers and Thomas Cadwalader. William Shippen, Sr., and John Redman were Presbyterians while Adam Kuhn was Lutheran, and John Morgan and the Bond brothers were Anglican.

10. Brooke Hindle, *The Pursuit of Science in Revolutionary America, 1735–1789* (Chapel Hill, N.C., 1956), 127–128; Bell, *John Morgan, Continental Doctor*, 122.

11. Bell, *John Morgan, Continental Doctor*, 124, 125, 137, 141, 157, 158.

12. Minutes, Oct. 23, 1793, St. George's Archives, London. Thomas Cadwalader and John Redman, for example, served as a team for twenty-five years. During the mid-1770's, Thomas Bond and William Shippen, Sr., worked together while newcomer John Morgan teamed up with newcomer Adam Kuhn.

13. Thomas Bond seemed to be the most charitably disposed in this sense. Bd. of M.M., I, II, passim.

14. Bond to Rhoads, London, December 20, 1771, Bond Autograph Collection, Philadelphia College of Physicians.

15. Morton and Woodbury, *History of the Pennsylvania Hospital*, 367–370. The physicians of the Almshouse were expected to supply medicine without any extra charge. Croskey, *History of Blockley*, 19.

16. Croskey, *History of Blockley*, 13. For proof that hagiography is not dead see accounts of physicians found throughout Morton and Woodbury, *History of the Pennsylvania Hospital* and Francis Packard, *Some Account of the Pennsylvania Hospital*.

17. Thacher, *American Medical Biography*, 179. Bd. of M.M., I, 63, 222. For other examples of Thomas Bond performing lithotomies (surgical incisions of the urinary bladder for removal of a stone) see Bd. of M.M., II, 127, 315–316, 400; III, 159. John Jones is often given credit for the first lithotomy in the colonies but Elizabeth Thomson maintains that Thomas Bond was first. Thomson,

"Thomas Bond, 1713–1784," *Journal of Medical Education*, XXXIII, no. 9 (1958), 622. For support of Miss Thomson's position note also Norris, *Early History of Medicine in Philadelphia*, 25.

18. Bell, *John Morgan, Continental Doctor*, 30–43, 125–127. There is nothing in the Hospital Archives to contradict this assumption.

19. Bd. of M.M., II, 127, 130.

20. My evidence is impressionistic on this count. Elizabeth Thomson first suggested to me the relationship of Thomas Bond's membership on the admission committees (two physicians and two Managers served) and the number of mental patients admitted at that time. After going through the Admission Committee Reports, also called Attending Managers Accounts, Pennsylvania Hospital Archives, I feel that the above statement is a fair one.

21. Bd. of M.M., I, 92, 93.

22. *Ibid.*, II, 25; IV, 71, 72.

23. *Ibid.*, IV, 78, 304. According to the Bd. of M.M., the "rules concerning choice and regulation of physicians at the Pennsylvania Hospital" adopted in 1752, provided that students pay a standard fee but evidently this regulation was not carried out. Bd. of M.M., I, 41.

24. Pemberton to Fothergill, June 30, 1762, Pemberton Copy Book, 1740–1780, Pemberton Papers, 219, Historical Society of Pennsylvania.

25. Bd. of M.M., II, 373, 378, 379, 414; III, 159, 163, 169, 181, 273; IV, 72, 314.

26. Fothergill to Pemberton, London, April 7, 1762, Etting-Pemberton Papers, Pemberton Papers, II, 47, Historical Society of Pennsylvania; Bd. of M.M., II, 325–327, 373, 374. The gift from Fothergill, contained in three shipping cases, was composed of "eighteen different parts of the human body in crayons framed and glaized, three cases of anatomical castings and one case containing a skeleton and foetus." The sketches were the works of Jan van Riemsdyk, a Dutch painter living in London with a considerable reputation in anatomical drawings. Bd. of M.M., II, 327; John W. Hoffman, "Jan van Riemsdyk," *Journal of American Medical Association*, April 7, 1969, 121. Fothergill's gift can be seen today in the Library of the Pennsylvania Hospital. Due to William Shippen, Jr.'s, interest in obstetrics, probably many of his lectures dealt with obstetrics. Morton and Woodbury, *History of the Pennsylvania Hospital*, 458.

27. Bd. of M.M., II, 326; Shryock, *The Development of Modern Medicine*, 38.

28. Norris, *The Early History of Medicine in Philadelphia*, 24; Bd. of M.M., IV, 72, 78.

29. Bell, *John Morgan, Continental Doctor*, 143–146; Bd. of M.M., III, 276–291.

30. Bd. of M.M., III, 276–291. Bond's introductory lectures can also be found in Morton and Woodbury's, *History of the Pennsylvania Hospital*, 462–467, and in Carl Bridenbaugh, "Dr. Thomas Bond's Essay on the Utility of Clinical Lectures," *Journal of the History of Medicine and Allied Sciences*, II (1949), 10–19. Shryock, *The Development of Modern Medicine*, 65; Bell, *John Morgan, Continental Doctor*, 90.

31. Bell, *John Morgan, Continental Doctor*, 146. For student complaints in 1774 against Thomas Bond's clinical lectures see *Ibid.*, 157. For praise see Thomson, "Thomas Bond, 1713–84," *Journal of Medical Education*, XXXIII, no. 9 (1958), 621.

32. William G. Malin, Sketch of the History of the Medical Library of the Pennsylvania Hospital, 4, 6, Historical Society of Pennsylvania; Bd. of M.M., II, 314, 379; III, 402, 297; IV, 94, 304, 325, 326; Whitfield Bell, Jr., "The Old Library of the Pennsylvania Hospital," *Bulletin of the Medical Library Association*, Oct., 1972, 543–545.

33. Bd. of M.M., I, 236; IV, 160. The idea of charging a fee was John Fothergill's. See Bd. of M.M., II, 327.

34. *Ibid.*, I, 158, 66.

35. *Ibid.*, 157, 197; II, 54. John Morgan's more "advantageous" business prospect

was the position of regimental surgeon of Pennsylvania Provincial troops. See Bell, *John Morgan, Continental Doctor*, 30.

36. Bd. of M.M., II, 113, 114, 133, 141, 154, 158, 182.

37. *Pennsylvania Chronicle and Universal Advertizer*, July 11, 1768; *Pennsylvania Gazette*, September 3, 1767; Bd. of M.M., III, 407, 378, 394, 395. Weed was demanding a salary increase from £70 to £80 even though his wife, the matron of the Hospital, was no longer alive to earn her part of what had been a joint salary.

38. Bd. of M.M., III, 481, 407; IV, 21, 9.

39. *Ibid.*, IV, 18, 22.

40. *Ibid.*, 73, 74, 96, 225, 249, 250, 328, 371, 401; Maurice B. Gordon, *Aesculapius Comes to the Colonies* (Ventnor, N.J., 1949), 468. For more on James Hutchinson see Whitfield Bell, Jr., "James Hutchinson (1752–1793): a Physician in Politics," in *Medicine, Science and Culture*, eds., Lloyd G. Stevenson and Robert P. Multauf (Baltimore, 1968), 265–283.

41. Morton and Woodbury, *History of the Pennsylvania Hospital*, 480; Bd. of M.M., IV, 203, 254. Actually there were only two apprentices to the apothecary during the colonial period and one, Jacob Ehrenzeller, is listed as a medical apprentice by Morton and Woodbury. However, the Bd. of M.M. indicate that Ehrenzeller's training was, at first, to be taken under the Hospital's apothecary. Bd. of M.M., IV, 203.

42. See chapter 2, 49; Morton and Woodbury, *History of the Pennsylvania Hospital*, 544; Bd. of M.M., II, 22. Elizabeth Gardner's salary also included board and room for herself and her two children. Bd. of M.M., II, 75, 133, 186.

43. Bd. of M.M., III, 297, 407.

44. *Ibid.*, 313, 314, 477, 481, 494.

45. *Ibid.*, 494; IV, 212, 213, 225, 226, 317, 375, 383.

46. For a brief description of the evolution of the steward's responsibilities in the British Hospital from the seventeenth to the mid-nineteenth century, see Courtney Dainton, *The Story of England's Hospitals* (Springfield, Ill., 1967), E. M. McIness, *St. Thomas Hospital* (Springfield, Ill., n.d.), 26, 27.

47. Bd. of M.M., II, 16.

48. *Ibid.*, 133, 62, 74.

49. *Ibid.*, 184. In England, during the eighteenth century, hospital matrons were slowly losing their authority. Shryock, *History of Nursing*, 217.

50. Bd. of M.M., IV, 380. From July 14, 1769, to May 16, 1770, there was no steward.

51. The steward's salary is derived from subtracting matron Sarah Harlan's salary from the joint salary of John and Sophia Saxton (i.e. £75 minus £30). For an example of salaries in a comparable British voluntary hospital see J. Delpratt Harris, *Royal Devon and Exeter Hospital* (Exeter, 1922), 45.

52. Bd. of M.M., I, 23, 47, 55, 57, 60, 66; II, 183; IV, 217, 273. In the original contract that he signed, Motley waived the right to collect any back salary owed him by the Hospital if he misbehaved. The Board of Managers, while maintaining that Motley had "forfeited any just claim to any pay . . .," did consent to pay 50 shillings to Motley's wife after "his wife representing their necessitious circumstances and his incapacity to work," asked for help. Bd. of M.M., I, 68.

53. On Cell Keeper, Arthur Barker, received £36 per year in 1762; but his responsibilities went beyond that of cell keeper. Bd. of M.M., II, 277.

54. Bd. of M.M., I, 142; Shryock, *History of Nursing*, 231, n.

55. Bd. of M.M., I, 23, 44, 178; II, 208, 250, 336; IV, 136, 145; Harris, *The Royal Devon and Exeter Hospital*, 45.

56. Shryock, *History of Nursing*, 231; Bd. of M.M., I, 144; II, 189; III, 379.

57. Bd. of M.M., I, 181, 213, 234; II, 67, 70. No indication exists that any of the other nurses had previous hospital experience elsewhere before entering the service of the Pennsylvania Hospital.

58. *Ibid.*, I, 178, 181. During th 1760's, the number of nurses never exceeded two and sometimes only one was employed at a time. In the 1770's, however, the records indicate that three nurses working simultaneously was the norm.

59. *Ibid.*, I, 142; II, 118, 136; IV, 136, 145; II, 336. In May of 1773, the accounts of the Hospital listed four nurses on the payroll. Bd. of M.M., IV, 228.

60. Bd. of M.M., I, 150, 160; II, 118, 136. The generalization concerning the 1760's and 1770's are based on the examination of the steward's monthly reports in the Bd. of M.M. for that period plus a scanning of the Steward's Cash Books for that same period. It is often difficult to separate nurses from maids because the records often use only their names and omit their titles. Thus I have often differentiated the maids from the nurses on the basis of salary.

61. Again this is a summary of sources too numerous to cite but found in the matron's and steward's reports in Bd. of M.M., and in the Matron's and Steward's Cash Books for the colonial period. The one mention that I have uncovered of an indentured servant employed as a maid is found in Bd. of M.M., IV, 197. For an example of salaries paid provincial hospital maids in Great Britain see Harris, *The Royal Devon and Exeter Hospital*, 45.

62. Bd. of M.M., III, 530, 531. The washerwoman and carpenter citations appear often in the Bd. of M.M. and, therefore, I have not bothered to cite them.

63. George Roberts Smith, Summary of Fiscal History of Hospital, Pennsylvania Hospital Archives, not paginated. Liancourt, *Travels Through the U.S. of North America*, 93, 94. The exceeding of one hundred poor patients at a time occurred most commonly during the last ten years of the colonial period. Bd. of M.M., I-V; Attending Managers Accounts, Pennsylvania Hospital Archives, 1770–1776. The Attending Managers Accounts must be used to supplement the Bd. of M.M. for the period 1770–1776, because the Bd. of M.M. ceases to list patients according to "poor" or "pay" categories after the middle of 1770.

64. Bd. of M.M., I, 38, 40, 47, 97, 99; II, 86, 331.

65. One might suspect that the use of one month—in this case April—as an indicator of how many patients were in residence throughout the year may be misleading. It could be argued, for example, that the number of patients in residence fluctuated greatly according to the seasons. To counteract this charge I have compiled a listing of patients in residence at the Hospital throughout the year from 1775, 1760, 1765, 1770 and 1775. The figures indicate that there is no clear seasonal pattern to the number of patients in the Hospital at a given time.

Patients in Residence at the Pennsylvania Hospital
(based on information in Bd. of M.M., I-V;
and
Attending Managers' Accounts, 1770–1775)

	1775	1760	1765	1770	1775
January	12	41	124	131	108
February	16	38	125	131	106
March	16	42	127	120	106
April	20	40	115	114	95
May	17	46	108	111	96
June	14	41	110	108	93
July	17	41	113	109	95
August	18	46	114	117	78
September	20	46	127	117	97
October	15	46	123	122	97
November	15	40	117	117	107
December	15	45	117	121	83

66. Resident figures of patients for the month of April.

	Total	Insane		Total	Insane
1755	20	5	1766	115	37
1756	19	2	1767	103	33
1757	24	5	1768	111	38
1758	27	10	1769	98	33
1759	36	10	1770	114	38
1760	41	16	1771	116	37
1761	43	15	1772	105	31
1762	52	25	1773	102	36
1763	76	23	1774	111	40
1764	99	37	1775	95	24
1765	115	34	1776	62	19

Based on Bd. of M.M., I-V, and Attending Managers' Accounts, 1770–1776.

67. Morton and Woodbury, *History of the Pennsylvania Hospital*, 240; Bd. of M.M., I-V; Attending Managers' Accounts 1770–1776; Turner, *The Story of a Great Hospital*, 93, 97, 98.

Number of Paying Patients in April for Selected Years

April	Total Lunatics	Total Lunatic Paying Patients	Total Paying Patients
1755	5	2	4
1760	16	7	15
1765	34	12	21
1770	38	12	19
1775	29	6	11

68. The raw figures on which the per diem costs are based were derived from Smith, Summary of Fiscal History of Hospital, Pennsylvania Hospital Archives, not paginated. The method used was to divide the average number of patients on a given date X 365 days into the total Hospital expenses for the year. The expense of building the new Hospital on Eighth and Pine was not included in the calculation of the Hospital's expenses. As mentioned previously, all financial statements are in terms of Pennsylvania currency unless otherwise indicated.

69. Bd. of M.M., II, 210, 211, 441; III, 9; IV, 340.

70. *Ibid.*, II, 73; IV, 72, 193, 207, 308; II, 210, 254, 440; III, 128.

71. *Ibid.*, II, 73, 79.

72. See, for example, James, *A People Among Peoples*, chapters VII, XII.

73. Bd. of M.M., II, 118, 318, 404.

74. The percentage of venereal patients housed in the Hospital in 1767 is based on listings of individual patients for 1767, Bd. of M.M., III, 321–347. Because this listing does not differentiate between "poor" and "pay" patients it is difficult to ascertain how many or what percentage of the venereal patients would be affected by the five shilling increase in the weekly rate. Bd. of M.M., III, 425.

75. The percentage of venereal patients housed in the Hospital in 1769 is based on the listing for individual patients for 1769. Bd. of M.M., III, 557–586.

76. Based on summary in Morton and Woodbury, *History of the Pennsylvania Hospital*, 240 and yearly reports in Bd. of M.M.

77. Bd. of M.M., I, 113, 188; IV, 308, 368, 422.

78. *Ibid.*, I, 37.

79. Morton and Woodbury, *History of the Pennsylvania Hospital*, 275, 283, 287.

80. Robert Honyman, *Colonial Panorama, 1775*, ed., Philip Padelford (San Marino, Calif., 1939), 15, 16; Andrew Burnaby, *Travels Through North America, 1759–1760*, ed., R. R. Wilson (New York, 1904), 90; *Pennsylvania Gazette*, February 28, 1771.

81. Attending Managers Accounts, February 25, 1775, May 25, 1775; Adams, *The Adams Papers, Diary and Autobiography of John Adams,* ed., Butterfield, II, 150.

82. Although the New York Hospital was founded in 1773, it was not really functioning as intended until after the Revolutionary War.

83. Carl and Jessica Bridenbaugh, *Rebels and Gentlemen,* 244–247. Bridenbaugh does not list, with the exception of John Adams, the names of the "visitors" who praised the Hospital. Therefore, I am not sure, with the exception of Adams, who these "visitors" were.

84. Shryock, *The History of Nursing,* 180, 181; Treasurer's Cash Book, July 11, 1764, and passim.

85. Morton and Woodbury, *History of the Pennsylvania Hospital,* 127–129; Bd. of M.M., II, 269.

86. Bd. of M.M., I, 140; II, 23, 34, 113; IV, 257; III, 65.

87. *Ibid.,* II, 114, 153, 178, 379; Morton and Woodbury, *History of the Pennsylvania Hospital,* 134.

88. *Ibid.,* I, 113; II, 120, 153; Treasurer's Cash Book, Feb. 28, 1764, 49.

89. Matron's Cash Book, passim; Steward's Cash Book, passim; Dainton, *The Story of England's Hospitals,* 80, 81; Bd. of M.M., II, 112, 133; III, 374, 425.

90. Bd. of M.M., III, 31, 164, supports the statement that Bibles and other religious materials were available for reading. The rest of the paragraph is conjecture based on impressions gathered from a number of scattered sources.

91. Bd. of M.M., II, 333; III, 22. The number of jailed criminals admitted to the Hospital was quite small as only a couple of clear references are made.

92. Boorstin, *The Americans, The Colonial Experience,* 237; Bridenbaugh, *Rebels and Gentlemen,* 246, 247. Boorstin's generalization is based on faulty figures which he probably borrowed (incorrectly at that) from Carl and Jessica Bridenbaugh's *Rebels and Gentlemen,* 246, 247. Professor Bridenbaugh maintains that the Pennsylvania Hospital admitted 8,831 patients from its founding until 1777, while Boorstin uses the same figure to represent admissions up to 1773. However, a check of the Bd. of M.M., Morton and Woodbury, *History of the Pennsylvania Hospital,* 240, and George Roberts Smith's Summary of Fiscal History of Hospital, not paginated, indicate that the total number of admissions during this period (1753–1777) was about 6,550. This revised figure makes a big difference in figuring the mortality rate for patients admitted to the Pennsylvania Hospital.

93. See, for example, J. H. Woodward, "Before Bacteriology—Deaths in Hospitals," *Yorkshire Faculty Journal,* Autumn, 1969, 1–10; E. M. Sigsworth, "A Provincial Hospital in the Eighteenth and Early Nineteenth Centuries," *Yorkshire Faculty Journal,* June, 1966, 24–31; Hyslop, London Hospitals in the Eighteenth Century, 70–72. My own research into British hospital records supports this revisionist view. *The History and Statutes of the Royal Infirmary of Edinburgh* (Edinburgh, 1749), 14; *The History and Statutes of the Royal Infirmary of Edinburgh* (Edinburgh, 1778), 29; Susan Fairclough, The Royal Infirmary of Edinburgh, 1770–1775, an unpublished paper in archives of the Royal Infirmary of Edinburgh, table in back; Synopsis of Patients, Quarterly Account, 34, not paginated, Records of the Devon and Exeter Hospital, Devon Records Office, Exeter Devonshire. The Rev. P. Doddridge, *Compassion to the Sick Recommended and Urged* (London, 1743), 25, notes that up to 1743, figures received from the infirmaries at Winchester, Bath, Exeter, York, Bristol, London and Westminster, indicate that some 7,330 patients are known cured and only 784 have died or been discharged as incurable.

94. Bd. of M.M., I-IV, passim.

95. Raw figures for this statement on the insane from 1759 to 1763 are found in Bd. of M.M., II, 109, 110, 175, 176, 238, 239, 298, 299, 370, 371.

96. Bd. of M.M., I, 41.

97. Boorstin, *The Americans, The Colonial Experience,* 214.

Chapter 4

1. James, *A People Among Peoples,* 244–246.

2. Raw figures for these yearly averages were found in George Roberts Smith, Summary of Fiscal History of Hospital, 1846, not paginated. According to Theodore Thayer, *Israel Pemberton,* 226, 227, some of the Quakers, including Hospital Manager Israel Pemberton and Owen Jones who would become a Manager in 1781, were not above exchanging gold for paper currency at an advantageous rate.

3. Hinshaw, *Encyclopedia of American Quaker Geneology,* II, passim; Scharf and Westcott, *History of Philadelphia,* III, 2275.

4. Thayer, *Israel Pemberton,* 203, 204, 207; Scharf and Westcott, *History of Philadelphia,* I, 290. For a detailed study of Quaker attitudes towards the Revolutionary War, see Arthur J. McKell, The Society of Friends (Quakers) and the American Revolution (Ph.D. dissertation, Harvard University, 1940).

5. Thayer, *Israel Pemberton,* 210–214.

6. Bd. of M.M., IV, 372, 426, 428, 439.

7. *Colonial Records,* XI, 34, 85, 130; Bd. of M.M., IV, 445–448; V, 5, 29, 33; Scharf and Westcott, *History of Philadelphia,* I, 335; James, *A People Among Peoples,* 245.

8. Bd. of M.M., V, 37, 39, 41, 140.

9. *Ibid.,* 43, 45, 59, 297; Scharf and Westcott, *History of Philadelphia,* I, 373.

10. John Richard Alden, *The American Revolution; 1775 to 1783* (New York, 1954), 112–126, 194–205; Howard H. Peckham, *The War for Independence; A Military History* (Chicago, 1958), 68–73, passim; Scharf and Westcott, *History of Philadelphia,* I, 350, 433.

11. Isaac Sharpless, *A History of Quaker Government in Pennsylvania,* II (Philadelphia, 1899), 160; Bd. of M.M., V, 37, 90; Scharf and Westcott, *History of Philadelphia,* I, 346; Thayer, *Israel Pemberton,* 229, 231.

12. Bd. of M.M., V, 73, 85, 86, 79.

13. Sharpless, *A History of Quaker Government in Pennsylvania,* II, 172; James, *A People Among Peoples,* 246, 247.

14. Morton and Woodbury, *History of the Pennsylvania Hospital,* 60; Bd. of M.M., V, 76, 90–93, 156. The Elaboratory was rented to the Continental Army at £50 per year. Getting the United States Government to pay the rent was, however, another question. In September of 1782 Manager Reynold Keene reported that although his committee "for obtaining rent due for the Elaboratory" had made frequent applications, it was not "as yet able to bring the matter to a favorable issue." Finally on September 29, 1783, Robert Morris agreed that the Hospital be paid £81.50, which represented "the full rent due" since he had become superintendent of finance for the United States. Bd. of M.M., V, 268, 277, 289, 325.

15. Thayer, *Israel Pemberton,* 214. One might argue that in 1776, when the Hospital accepted some Continental soldiers, the Hospital was cooperating openly with revolutionaries. It must be noted, however, that by admitting revolutionary soldiers the Hospital was merely obeying an order from the Council of Safety because there was no other choice without recourse to bloodshed. Adjutant General Bond's proposal, by contrast, was not an order but a request and therefore could be refused.

16. Bd. of M.M., V, 113, 121, 139, 140; Smith, Summary of Fiscal History of Hospital, not paginated; Robert Brunhouse, *Counter Revolution in Pennsylvania* (Harrisburg, Pa., 1942), 26; *Journals of the House of Representatives of the Commonwealth of Pennsylvania* (Philadelphia, 1782), 454. After the war the Hospital presented a bill to the state for medical services rendered certain soldiers. The state, however, maintained that the £10,000 grant was a loan and that it could be used to pay the claim. After an appeal by the Board, the Assembly officially made the loan a gift. For an idea of how worthless continental paper money

was in Philadelphia by 1779, see costs of specific items mentioned in Scharf and Westcott, *History of Philadelphia*, II, 901.

17. Smith, Summary of Fiscal History of Hospital, not paginated; Morton and Woodbury, *History of the Pennsylvania Hospital*, 249. The total sum from prize money received by the Hospital amounted to about £2,300.

18. Bd. of M.M., V, 291, 294; Morton and Woodbury, *History of the Pennsylvania Hospital*, 249.

19. Hinshaw, *Encyclopedia of American Quaker Geneology*, II, passim. Eleven of the twenty "new" Managers were Quakers. Morton and Woodbury, *History of the Pennsylvania Hospital*, 414–421.

20. Hinshaw, *Encyclopedia of American Quaker Geneology*, II, passim; Morton and Woodbury, *History of the Pennsylvania Hospital*, 487; Tolles, *Meeting House and Counting House*, 226. For more details on the Shippen-Morgan dispute during the Revolution see Bell, *John Morgan, Continental Doctor*, chapters XI–XIII. For one reason why Rush did not care for Shippen see Bell, *John Morgan, Continental Doctor*, 157.

21. Attending Managers' Accounts, passim.

22. Bd. of M.M., V, 298, 312, 318; Bell, *John Morgan, Continental Doctor*, 241, 242. For documentation of how hard Thomas Bond worked for the Hospital during the Revolutionary years see Attending Managers Accounts, passim. From November, 1777, through March, 1778, Thomas Bond was the lone physician in attendance at the Hospital. From October, 1778, through February, 1779, he again performed as the only physician in attendance at the Hospital. The relationship between the House of Employment and the Pennsylvania Hospital will be dealt with in Chapter V.

23. Henry Simpson, *The Lives of Eminent Philadelphians* (Philadelphia, 1859), 158; Bell, "James Hutchinson (1752–1793): Letters from an American Student in London," *Transactions and Studies of College of Physicians of Philadelphia*, 4th ser., XXXIV, 20–23; Morton and Woodbury, *History of the Pennsylvania Hospital*, 491–493; Attending Managers Minutes, 1778, 1779. Shippen's failure to serve the Hospital during the year 1778–1779, is understandable in view of his position of Director General of the Continental Hospital. James Hutchinson left the Hospital after only one year's service to join the army as a surgeon. In 1779 he returned to the Hospital staff and continued to serve the Hospital until his death in 1793.

24. *Pennsylvania Journal and Weekly Advertiser*, May 1, 1782; Bd. of M.M., V, 5, 85, 144, 192, 217, 164, 271, 284, 338; Morton and Woodbury, *History of the Pennsylvania Hospital*, 533, 543. I am grateful to George H. M. Lawrence of East Greenwich, R.I. for information on Kiellman.

25. *Ibid.*, IV, 375, 383; V, 67, 79, 127, 130. Evidently the Board had been fairly well pleased with John Story because, after Story left the Hospital, he was given a bonus of £16. Bd. of M.M., V, 146.

26. *Ibid.*, V, 133, 136, 192, 194, 223, 236, 286.

27. *Ibid.*, V, 47; IV, 423; V, 96, 220.

28. The above statistics are found in Bd. of M.M., IV–VII; Rough Minutes, 1781–1784; Liancourt, *Travels Through the U.S. of North America*, 93, 94.

29. Statistics for the insane patients were found by counting individually each patient still in residence at the end of April of each year. Bd. of M.M., IV–VII and Rough Minutes, 1775–1783.

30. This is part speculation as the relevant figures are hard to dig out. However, an examination of figures from 1755, 1760, 1765, 1770, 1775 support this generalization. Bd. of M.M., I–IV; Attending Managers Accounts, 1771–1775.

31. Attending Managers Accounts, 1779, 1783; Bd. of M.M., V, 186.

32. Bd. of M.M., I, 113, 188; IV, 308, 368, 422; V, 76, 111.

33. *Ibid.*, V, 37, 43, 67, 74, 81, 86, 111, 126, 144, 166, 190, 195, 217, 220, 228, 234.

34. *Ibid.*, IV, 248, 302, 366, 422; V, 25, 65, 109, 163, 211, 262, 311. The figures

cited do not include military personnel who were housed at the Hospital during
the Revolution. The British sick and wounded were not recorded but the Hospital did record that 129 Continental soldiers, seamen and Hessian prisoners were
admitted and 28 died. Bd. of M.M., V, 22–25, 258–262.

Chapter 5

1. James, *A People Among Peoples*, 290, 291.
2. Moreau de St. Méry, *Moreau de St. Méry's American Journey*, eds. and trans.
Kenneth Roberts and Anna M. Roberts (Garden City, N.Y., 1947), 357; Charles
Lawrence, *History of the Philadelphia Almshouses and Hospitals* (Philadelphia,
1905), 36; Edward P. Cheyney, *History of the University of Pennsylvania*
(Philadelphia, 1940), 176; Maynard Pressley White, An Account of the First
College Edifice of Washington College, 1783–1827 (an unpublished master's
thesis at Morris Library, University of Delaware), 128 and passim. Obviously
there were some exceptions to the above generalization.
3. These statistics were compiled from a variety of sources with Morton and Woodbury, *History of the Pennsylvania Hospital*, and Hinshaw, *Encyclopedia of
American Quaker Geneology*, II, being most helpful.
4. The generalization that the Managers continued to come primarily from the
mercantile community is based on a sample group of fifteen Managers who were
examined. Information on their vocations came primarily from Morton and
Woodbury, *History of the Pennsylvania Hospital;* John W. Jordan, ed., *Colonial
Families of Philadelphia*, Henry Simpson, *Lives of Eminent Philadelphians Now
Deceased* (Philadelphia, 1859), and Stephen Noyes Winslow, *Biographies of
Successful Philadelphia Merchants* (Philadelphia, 1864).
5. Information on Samuel Coates is found primarily in the manuscript collection of
the Historical Society of Pennsylvania; Henry Simpson, *Lives of Eminent Philadelphians*, 212–228; Morton and Woodbury, *History of the Pennsylvania Hospital*, 421, 422; Winslow, *Biographies of Successful Philadelphia Merchants*, 192–
195. From 1786 until 1823 he served as one of "The Overseers of the Public
Schools, founded by charter in the town and county of Philadelphia." From
1800 until its demise in 1811, Coates was a director of the First Bank of the
United States.
6. Morton and Woodbury, *History of the Pennsylvania Hospital*, 139–142, 152, 153,
421; Bd. of M.M., VI, 78, 273, 389.
7. Morton and Woodbury, *History of the Pennsylvania Hospital*, 420, 421, 423;
Winslow, *Biographies of Successful Philadelphia Merchants*, 230–233; Bd. of
M.M., VI, passim. I have uncovered no information to indicate that Josiah
Hewes was a Quaker.
8. Pemberton to Fothergill, Philadelphia, October 14, 1779, Pemberton Copy Book,
1740–1780, 286, Historical Society of Pennsylvania; Johann David Schoepf,
Travels in the Confederation (1783–1784), trans. and ed., Alfred J. Morrison
(Philadelphia, 1911), 70, 71.
9. Smith, Summary of Fiscal History of Hospital, Pennsylvania Hospital Archives,
not paginated. It must be pointed out that the £722 was not necessarily the
income from one year as it could have included late rent and interest payments
from past years.
10. Bd. of M.M., VI, 14, 59, 78, 82, 107, 113, 121. No doubt liquor was used to
tranquilize some of the insane patients.
11. *Ibid.*, 65, 269; Smith, Summary of Fiscal History of Hospital, not paginated.
12. Bd. of M.M., VI, 14, 20; Smith, Summary of Fiscal History of Hospital, not
paginated.
13. Bd. of M.M., VI, 78, 109, 119, 144; Morton and Woodbury, *History of the
Pennsylvania Hospital*, 263, 267.
14. Anne Bezanson, *Prices and Inflation During the American Revolution, Pennsylvania 1770–1790* (Philadelphia, 1951), 10; Bd. of M.M., VI, 29, 30, 57.
15. Bd. of M.M., V, 307; VI, 256, 257; VII, 412.

170   America's First Hospital: The Pennsylvania Hospital, 1751–1841

16. *Ibid.,* VI, 107, 121, 277, 288, 369.

17. *Ibid.,* 67.

18. *Ibid.,* VII, 374, 87, 89, 92, 98.

19. Smith, Summary of Fiscal History of Hospital, not paginated; Bd. of M.M., VI, 505. Liancourt, after visiting the Hospital in 1797, supported the above generalizations by noting that "in 1775, the Hospital received seventy patients gratis; but, although its revenues are not diminished since that period, the increase of the price of provisions, and of the wages of the persons employed in the Hospital, is so great, that at present it can take no more than thirty patients gratis." Liancourt, *Travels Through the U.S. of North America,* IV, 2nd ed., 94.

20. Morton and Woodbury, *History of the Pennsylvania Hospital,* 279–287; Bd. of M.M., VI, 131, 137, 148, 151, 85, 111, 133, 268, 341; VII, 5.

21. J. P. Brissot de Warville, *New Travels in the U.S. of North America, 1788,* ed., Durand Echeverria (Cambridge, Mass., 1964), 179; Bd. of M.M., VI, 389.

22. Bd. of M.M., VI, 447, 448, 451, 455; VII, 92. Smith, Fiscal History of Hospital, not paginated. Morton and Woodbury, *History of the Pennsylvania Hospital,* 254.

23. Charles E. Peterson, "Carpenters Hall," *Historic Philadelphia: From the Founding Until the Early Nineteenth Century,* Luther Eisenhart, ed. (Philadelphia, 1953), 126; Peterson, "Library Hall," *Historic Philadelphia,* 135, 131, 143; Bd. of M.M., VI, 515. All statements transferring Pennsylvania pound values to dollars are based on equivalents found in Bd. of M.M.

24. Bd. of M.M., VI, 516, 519, 520.

25. *Ibid.,* VII, 6, 7, 57.

26. *Ibid.,* 32, 34, 73, 78, 79. The first payment from unclaimed bankruptcy dividends was not made to the Hospital until December 16, 1795, some three weeks after the Board requested aid from Governor Mifflin.

27. Bd. of M.M., VII, 94, 116, 151, 140; Morton and Woodbury, *History of the Pennsylvania Hospital,* 376, 255–262. Income from the Legislature's Loan Office Act of 1793 continued to be collected, however, until 1804. Morton and Woodbury, *History of the Pennsylvania Hospital,* 262.

28. Bd. of M.M., VII, 152, 195, 202, 213, 261, 327, 373; Morton and Woodbury, *History of the Pennsylvania Hospital,* 79.

29. Engraving of Library Hall is reproduced in Peterson, "Library Hall: Home of the Library Company of Philadelphia, 1790–1880," *Historic Philadelphia; From the Founding Until the Early Nineteenth Century,* ed. Luther Eisenhart, 129.

30. *Ibid.,* 132, 132 n., 133–135; Maynard Pressley White, Jr., An Account of the First College Edifice of Washington College (unpublished master's thesis, Morris Library, University of Delaware, 1966), 93. Significantly Joseph Paschall and Thomas Morris were on the Hospital's building committee.

31. *An Account of the Rise, Progress and Present State of the Pennsylvania Hospital* (Philadelphia, 1801), 5, 6; Bd. of M.M., VII, 213.

32. Charles Lawrence, *History of the Philadelphia Almshouses and Hospitals* (Philadelphia 1905), 20; John Welsh Croskey, ed., *History of Blockley: A History of the Philadelphia General Hospital from Its Inception, 1731–1928* (Philadelphia, 1929), 13; D. Hayes Agnew, "The Medical History of the Philadelphia Almshouse," ed. Croskey, *History of Blockley,* 18.

33. Franklin, *Some Account of the Pennsylvania Hospital,* ed. Cohen, 1, 4; Packard, *Some Account of the Pennsylvania Hospital,* 3–5; Morton and Woodbury, *History of the Pennsylvania Hospital,* 220.

34. Bridenbaugh, *Rebels and Gentlemen,* 247. Bridenbaugh does not give his source for this early date and D. Hayes Agnew, "The Medical History of the Philadelphia Almshouse," ed. John W. Croskey, *History of Blockley,* 18, 19, maintains that the earliest extant records on Almshouse physicians speak of doctors Thomas Bond and Cadwalader Evans being reappointed to the Almshouse staff in 1769. To further point out the medical differences between the two institutions the following facts should be noticed:

a. The Pennsylvania Hospital employed its first apothecary in 1752 but the Almshouse did not hire its first apothecary until 1788. Bd. of M.M., I, 66; Agnew (see above), 49.

b. From its inception the Pennsylvania Hospital contained cells for the insane but the Almshouse did not have cells constructed until 1803. Agnew (see above), 46.

c. Clinical lectures were formally introduced in the Pennsylvania Hospital in the winter of 1766–1767 while it was not until 1803 that the same practice went on in the Almshouse. Bd. of M.M., III, 276–291; Lawrence, *History of Philadelphia Almshouses and Hospitals*, 43.

d. Medical students were allowed to observe practice in the Pennsylvania Hospital from the very beginning but it was not until 1788 that they were admitted to the Almshouse. See Chapter 5; Lawrence, *History of Philadelphia Almshouses and Hospitals*, 35.

e. One of the significant developments in the evolution of the medieval hospital into the modern hospital was the decision to accept only curable patients. Arrived at in England during the seventeenth century, this decision helped distinguish between the evolving "modern" hospital and the almshouses which accepted everyone who was impoverished and incapable of providing for himself. The Pennsylvania Hospital followed the "modern" hospital tradition by accepting, except for some lunatics, only curable patients. By contrast, the Philadelphia Almshouse, as far as I can discern, was not discriminating in its admissions.

35. Bd. of M.M., VII, 172. Warville, *New Travels in the U.S. of North America, 1788*, ed. Echeverria, 173; Agnew, "The Medical History of the Philadelphia Almshouse," ed. Croskey, *History of Blockley*, 33.

36. Bridenbaugh, *Rebels and Gentlemen*, 233, 234; Lawrence, *History of Philadelphia Almshouses and Hospitals*, 22; *Colonial Records*, XI, 776; Warville, *New Travels in the U.S. of North America, 1788*, ed. Echeverria, 174. Rhoads, according to Bridenbaugh, *Rebels and Gentlemen*, 200, may have had an important role in the designing of the "new" Almshouse.

37. Morton and Woodbury, *History of the Pennsylvania Hospital*, 218; Bd. ofM. M., VI, 501, 233, 240, 369. Actually the suit was filed by the Hospital against the Guardians of the Poor, a body that had ultimate authority over the board of managers of the Almshouse. The Almshouse maintained that the Hospital had been set up to serve, exclusively, Pennsylvania's sick-poor. Therefore, it was illegal for the Hospital to admit nonpaying sick-poor who were foreigners or inhabitants of other states.

38. Bd. of M.M., VII, 308–310, 387; Lawrence, *History of Philadelphia Almshouses*, 49, 50. The Almshouse seemed to be able to handle most cases of disease at this time (last two decades of the eighteenth century) but admitted that the Pennsylvania Hospital was better equipped to handle venereal cases and lunatics.

39. Coates to Moses Brown, October 12, 1795, Samuel Coates Letter Book, 13, Historical Society of Pennsylvania; Lawrence, *History of the Philadelphia Almshouses*, 51.

Chapter 6

1. See *D.A.B.*, passim; Henry Simpson, *Lives of Eminent Philadelphians;* Howard A. Kelly and Walter Burrage, eds., *Dictionary of American Medical Biography* (New York, 1928). Only two Managers were listed in the *D.A.B.* who served during the "recovery period" (1784–1801). They were Samuel Coates and Robert Waln.

2. The five physicians who received Edinburgh degrees were Adam Kuhn, William Shippen, Jr., Philip Syng Physick, Caspar Wistar and Benjamin Rush. John Jones, Thomas Parke and Benjamin Smith Barton spent some time at Edinburgh, and Barton would have received his degree from that institution but refused because of "the discourteous manner in which two of the professors at the University of Edinburgh had treated him." James Hutchinson did not travel from London to Edinburgh because he was interested in the American Revolution and

in getting back to Philadelphia as soon as possible. Kelly and Burrage, eds., *Dictionary of American Medical Biography,* 68; Morton and Woodbury, *History of the Pennsylvania Hospital,* 491–498; Whitfield Bell, Jr., "James Hutchinson (1752–1793): A Physician in Politics," *Medicine, Science and Culture,* eds., Lloyd G. Stevenson and Robert P. Multhauf, 270–272.

3. John Adams to Thomas Jefferson, June 30, 1813, in *Adams-Jefferson Letters,* II, ed., Lester J. Cappon (Chapel Hill, N.C., 1959), 347.

4. Bd. of M.M., VI, 72; VII, 222, 374, 361.

5. *Ibid.,* VI, 501, 502.

6. Scharf and Westcott, *History of Philadelphia,* I, 480; Binger, *Revolutionary Doctor: Benjamin Rush, 1746–1813;* Correspondence of Dr. Benjamin Rush, Library Company Collection, XXXI, 34, Historical Society of Pennsylvania; Bd. of M.M., VI, 502.

7. The Rush-Kuhn acrimony probably began back in 1774 when Rush sided with Shippen and John Morgan in an attempt to halt Thomas Bond's clinical lectures. Kuhn rushed to the aid of Bond during this dispute (see Chapter 3). Later the two physicians (Rush and Kuhn) disagreed over proper therapy. This aspect of their clash, however, will be taken up later in this chapter. The clash between Wistar and Rush also probably concerned therapy but is only alluded to and not spelled out in Samuel Coates to Benjamin Rush, October 28, 1793, Correspondence of Dr. Benjamin Rush, XXXI, 53, Library Company Collection, Historical Society of Pennsylvania. Rush's clash with William Shippen, Jr., goes back to the Morgan-Shippen dispute already spoken of in Chapter 3.

8. William G. Malin, Sketch of the History of the Medical Library of the Pennsylvania Hospital, 6–9, Historical Society of Pennsylvania; Bd. of M.M., VI, 113, 345; Morton and Woodbury, *History of the Pennsylvania Hospital,* 347–349; *An Account of the Rise, Progress and Present State of the Pennsylvania Hospital* (Philadelphia, 1801), 7; Manasseh Cutler, *Life, Journals and Correspondence of Rev. Manasseh Cutler,* ed. W. P. Cutler, et al., I, 279. For library rules and regulations see Bd. of M.M., VI, 279–281. Sarah Zane was described as "a wealthy maiden lady who inherited an extensive and valuable library collected by her ancestors, the medical portion of which she bestowed upon the Hospital." Malin, Sketch . . ., 8. Actually, the Zane collection had once belonged to William Byrd of Westover. For details on this gift plus other detailed information on the Hospital's library see Whitfield Bell, Jr., The Old Library of the Pennsylvania Hospital," *Bulletin of the Medical Library Association,* October, 1972, 543–550.

9. Bd. of M.M., VI, 404, 465; Kelly and Burrage, eds., *Dictionary of American Medical Biography,* 223, 224. The Hospital paid a life annuity of £50 or £30 (there is a disagreement between sources) to Abraham Chovet's widow in return for the preparations and wax models. In 1801 the collection in the anatomical museum (Chovet's and the others) was valued at $3,000. *An Account of the Rise, Progress and Present State of the Pennsylvania Hospital,* 7.

10. Bd. of M.M., VI, 444, 381, 82.

11. *Ibid.,* 138, 183, 374, 311, 312; Morton and Woodbury, *History of the Pennsylvania Hospital,* 480–481, 535. The indentured student received only his meals and shelter during his residency and thus had to depend on some outside source for clothes and other essentials. A bond was also posted to insure that the apprentice served out the years of the indenture. Bd. of M.M., VI, 107, 314.

12. Bd. of M.M., VII, 26, 328, 329; Morton and Woodbury, *History of the Pennsylvania Hospital,* 479, 480. Edward Cutbush later became an outstanding physician for the U.S. Navy (see Kelly and Burrage, eds., *Dictionary of American Medical Biography*).

13. Bd. of M.M., VI, 381. Hospital physicians on the medical school faculty of the University of Pennsylvania prior to 1801 included: Benjamin Smith Barton—professor of materia medica; John Foulke—lecturer on anatomy; James Hutchinson—professor of materia medica and chemistry; Adam Kuhn—professor of theory and practice of medicine; Benjamin Rush—professor of medical and clinical prac-

tices; William Shippen, Jr.—professor of anatomy, mid-wifery and surgery; and Caspar Wistar—adjunct professor of anatomy, mid-wifery and surgery.

14. Morton and Woodbury, *History of the Pennsylvania Hospital,* 532–535; Bd. of M.M., V, 341; VI, 1, 49, 53, 195. Due to the American Revolution, the Pennsylvania Hospital was forced to turn to domestic sources for its wholesale purchases of drugs. Once the Revolution had ended the new pattern continued because American wholesale firms were expanding their activities and even beginning to venture into the business of manufacturing pharmaceutical chemicals on a large scale. See Edward Kremmers and George Urdung, *History of Pharmacy,* 2nd ed. (Philadelphia, 1952), 221, 222, 247.

15. Bd. of M.M., VI, 82, 107.

16. *Ibid.,* VI, 381, 392; VII, 64, 87, 506. Mary Falconer later reappeared in the employment of the Hospital as nurse of the venereal disease ward during the later 1790's.

17. *An Account of the Rise, Progress and Present State of the Pennsylvania Hospital* (Philadelphia, 1801), 6; Steward's Cash Books, passim. The above generalizations concerning the number of employees is correct in an approximate sense. The Steward's Cash Books list each of the positions mentioned in its account of salaries paid out, but these references are scattered at best and therefore generalizations based on them may not be exact on a given date. The number of nurses and nurse's assistants, for example, seemed to fluctuate between three and six at any given time.

18. The above facts concerning the cell keepers have been gleaned from over fifty entries in both the Bd. of M.M., the Steward's Accounts; and the Steward's Cash Books for the years 1783–1801.

19. All of the above statements concerning nurses are taken from over a hundred citations in Bd. of M.M., 1783–1801, the Steward's Reports; and Steward's Cash Books for the same period. Generalizations concerning salaries of the stewards and cell keepers are based on the same sources.

20. As in footnotes 18 and 19, the sources are too numerous to list. Some seventy-five specific citations are the basis of generalizations and are found primarily in Bd. of M.M., 1783–1801, Steward's Reports and Steward's Cash Books for the same period. The history of early American nursing is an area that seems relatively untouched. Therefore it is difficult to make generalizations about American nurses of this era outside of the Pennsylvania Hospital.

21. Again the citations are too numerous to list. Some forty-one entries found in the Bd. of M.M., and Steward's Cash Books are the basis for the above statements. Often the Hospital hired part time employees to do odd jobs as well as to perform specialized services. Among these part time employees was one Richard Allen, who was probably the same black man who was a great friend of Benjamin Rush and founder of the African Methodist Episcopal Church. Bd. of M.M., VII, 162.

22. Whitfield Bell, Jr., "Social History of Pennsylvania, 1760–1790," *Pennsylvania Magazine of History and Biography,* LXII, 302; Benjamin Rish, *Letters of Benjamin Rush,* I, ed., L. H. Butterfield (Princeton, 1951), 448; Binger, *Revolutionary Doctor; Benjamin Rush,* 174. The Hospital figures for the five-year period are "probable" because records of the number of out-patients for this period are not extant. However, a few citations in the later 1790's indicate that between two and three hundred out-patients were treated annually at the Pennsylvania Hospital. Therefore, the figures of about 1,800 patients for 1787–1792 include approximately 1,250 (250 per year) out-patients.

23. Bd. of M.M., VII, 121, 260, 342; Benjamin Rush, *Letters of Benjamin Rush,* II, ed., Butterfield, 863.

24. Binger, *Revolutionary Doctor; Benjamin Rush,* 58; Kenneth and Anna Roberts, eds., *Moreau de St. Mery's American Journey* (New York, 1947), 354.

25. In his sampling of patients of the Pennsylvania Hospital, Robert W. Downie shows that the acceleration in the percentage of resident insane patients which

marked the post-war period (1783–1801) began to reverse itself by 1805. The Pennsylvania Hospital, however, continued to count insane patients as a majority of its resident patients until the removal of the insane patients to a new structure in West Philadelphia in 1841. Robert W. Downie, "Pennsylvania Hospital Admissions, 1751–1850; A Survey," *Transactions and Studies of the College of Physicians of Philadelphia*, XXXII (1964–65), 4th ser., 22.

26. Bd. of M.M., VII, passim; Downie, "Pennsylvania Hospital Admissions, 1751–1850: A Survey," *Transactions and Studies of the College of Physicians of Philadelphia*, XXXII (1964–1965), 22.

27. Albert Deutsch, *The Mentally Ill in America* (New York, 1949), 2nd ed., 65. Bethlehem ceased this practice in 1770. Johann David Schoepf, *Travels in the Confederation, 1783–1784*, ed. and trans., Alfred J. Morrison, 70; Bd. of M.M., VI, 10, 14, 373. Correspondence of Doctor Benjamin Rush, XXXI, 53, Library Company Collection, Historical Society of Pennsylvania.

28. Bd. of M.M., VI, 451. Brissot de Warville in his visit to the Hospital in 1788 was informed by Benjamin Rush that the "insane lodged immediately beneath the sick ward caused disturbances which woke the other patients in the middle of the night, thus delaying recovery." Warville, *New Travels in the U.S. of North America, 1788*, ed., Echeverria, 181.

29. Warville, *New Travels in the U.S. of North America*, ed., Echeverria, 179, 180; Rush, *Letters of Benjamin Rush*, ed., Butterfield, I, 528; Bd. of M.M., VII, 5. Circulating heated gases beneath the cell floor, a method which anticipated modern radiant heating, was introduced in the McLean Asylum, Waverly, Massachusetts, in 1826. But this type of development was both too late and too sophisticated to have been used by the Pennsylvania Hospital during the recovery period. Leonard K. Eaton, *New England Hospitals, 1790–1833* (Ann Arbor, Mich., 1957), 140.

30. Scharf and Westcott, *History of Philadelphia*, I, 499–501, 510; Correspondence of Doctor Benjamin Rush, XXXI, 53, Library Company Collection, Historical Society of Pennsylvania; Samuel Coates Letterbook, 46, Historical Society of Pennsylvania; David Gibson to ?, October 7, 1790, American Philosophical Society.

31. Liancourt, Travels through the U.S. of North America, 94; Rush, *Letters of Benjamin Rush*, ed., Butterfield, I, 529.

32. Warville, *New Travels in the U.S. of America, 1788*, ed., Echeverria, 179; Cutler, *Life, Journals, and Correspondence of Rev. Manasseh Cutler*, I, 280; Cecil Drinker, *Not So Long Ago* (New York, 1937), 28, 29; Bd. of M.M., VI, 335.

33. Bd. of M.M., VI, 49; VI, 127, 123; Steward's Cash Books, passim, April 24, 1790. Because the diet schedule of 1778 was drawn up when the Hospital was in dire financial straits, it was probably less nourishing than those used in peacetime and therefore should not be looked upon as entirely typical.

34. Hyslop, *London Hospitals in the Eighteenth Century*, 66; Turner, *Story of a Great Hospital*, 114.

35. James, *A People Among Peoples*, 271, Bd. of M.M., VI, 82; Steward's Cash Book, 1785–1792, passim. Benjamin Rush was convinced that excessive drinking of spirituous liquors was the cause of insanity of one half of the Hospital's lunatic patients. Liancourt, *Travels Through the U.S. of North America*, 95.

36. Bd. of M.M., VI, 507; Francis R. Packard, "Medical Case Histories in a Colonial Hospital," *Bulletin of the History of Medicine*, XII (1942), 145–168.

37. Binger, *Revolutionary Doctor, Benjamin Rush, 1746–1813*, 39, 228.

38. Elizabeth Thomson in "Thomas Bond, 1713–84," *Journal of Medical Education*, XXXIII, no. 9 (1958), 623, states that "in an age of drastic medical treatment, he (Thomas Bond) counseled moderation and common sense." In Chapter 3, n5, Thomas Cadwalader is shown to offer moderate therapy. Even John Redman, originally an advocate of extreme therapy, gave up excessive bleeding. Binger, *Revolutionary Doctor, Benjamin Rush, 1746–1813*, 228.

39. Rush, *Letters of Benjamin Rush*, ed., Butterfield, II, 759; Bell, "James Hutchin-

son, Physician in Politics," *Medicine, Science and Culture,* eds., Stevenson and Multhauf, 281; Drinker, *Not So Long Ago,* 151.

40. Rush, *Letters of Benjamin Rush,* ed. Butterfield, I, 443.

41. John Rush had previously earned a medical degree in 1804, only to forsake medicine for the U.S. Navy. The ostensible cause of John Rush's insanity was a duel in 1807 in which the younger Rush killed one of his best friends. In 1811, a melancholy Benjamin Rush wrote Thomas Jefferson that "he (John) is now in a cell in the Pennsylvania Hospital where there is too much reason that he will end his days." John Rush did "end his days" in the Hospital some twenty-seven years later. Binger, *Revolutionary Doctor, Benjamin Rush, 1746–1813,* 282, 283; Rush, *Letters of Benjamin Rush,* ed., Butterfield, II, 959, 960, n. The Polly Hefferman Story is found in Samuel Coates, The Memorandum Book of Samuel Coates, 35–38, Historical Library, Pennsylvania Hospital.

42. Deutsch, *The Mentally Ill in America,* 78, 79; Morton and Woodbury, *History of the Pennsylvania Hospital,* 163–165; Rush, *Letters of Benjamin Rush,* ed., Butterfield, I, 443, 766, 769, 784; Warville, *New Travels in the U.S. of America, 1788,* ed., Echeverria, 179. To further affect the blood circulation of insane patients Rush invented two mechanical devices called, respectively, the "tranquilizer" and the "gyrator." Deutsch, *The Mentally Ill in America,* 79; Morton and Woodbury, *History of the Pennsylvania Hospital,* 163, 164.

43. Pinel introduced a more humane treatment of the insane at the Bicêtre asylum in Paris in 1792. Tuke helped found the York Retreat in England, which opened its doors to the insane in 1796. At York as well as at Bicêtre, gentle or humane treatment was substituted for the harsh treatment traditionally given the insane. Deutsch, *The Mentally Ill in America,* 88–95.

44. Rush, *Letters of Benjamin Rush,* Butterfield, ed., II, 528, 529, 799, 1058, 1059.

45. Bd. of M.M., VII, 34; Deutsch, *The Mentally Ill in America,* 91, 94; Correspondence of Dr. Benjamin Rush, XXXIX, 146, Library Company Collection, Historical Society of Pennsylvania. Samuel Coates' Letterbook, Sept., 1795– May, 1802, 43, Historical Society of Pennsylvania.

46. The raw figures upon which the mortality summary and percentage was based are found in Bd. of M.M., V-VII, passim; Morton and Woodbury, *History of the Pennsylvania Hospital,* 242. Since the patient report for 1801 ended in April of that year, I also included 1802. Again, as for other periods in the Hospital's history, it might be argued that insane patients, because they remained in the Hospital longer than other patients would contribute to the high mortality rate. However, according to Benjamin Rush's own mortality figures for the years 1793 to 1802, mortality among the insane was certainly no higher than among the other patients. Correspondence of Doctor Benjamin Rush, XXXIX, 146, Library Company Collection, Historical Society of Pennsylvania.

Chapter 7

1. Gerald N. Grob, *Mental Institutions in America, Social Policy to 1875* (New York, 1973), 29, 30; Leonard K. Eaton, "Medicine in Philadelphia and Boston, 1805–1830," *Pennsylvania Magazine of History and Biography,* LXXV, 73; Eaton, *New England Hospitals, 1790–1833,* 84, passim. The only important early hospital that did not seem to have been influenced by the example of the Pennsylvania Hospital was what would be later known as the Eastern State Hospital, set up to receive "lunaticks," in Williamsburg, Virginia. The latter institution received its first patients in 1773. See Norman Dain, *Disordered Minds, The First Century of the Eastern State Hospital in Williamsburg, Virginia, 1766–1866* (Williamsburg, 1971).

2. Sam Bass Warner, *The Private City: Philadelphia in Three Periods of Its Growth* (Philadelphia, 1968), 51.

3. Bd. of M.M., VIII, 14–16, 185, 269, 362, 516; IX, 103. The official history was William G. Malin, *Some Account of the Pennsylvania Hospital, Its Origin, Objects and Present State* (Philadelphia, 1831).

4. See, for example, Grob, *Mental Institutions in America,* 64.

5. Bd. of M.M., VIII, 110, 122, 135, 203, 233–234, 236, 237, 244, 247, 254, 255; George B. Wood, *An Address on the Occasion of the Centennial Celebration of the Founding of the Pennsylvania Hospital* (Philadelphia, 1851), 36–38; Morton and Woodbury, *History of the Pennsylvania Hospital,* 294–303; W. I. Duane to Samuel Coates, March 12, 1814, Letter Book, Archives of Pennsylvania Hospital. *Journal of the House of Representatives of the Commonwealth of Pennsylvania, 1815, 1816* (Harrisburg, 1816), 277, 579, 698–700, 703. See also other letters from Samuel Coates to members of the state legislature in the Letter Book on the antagonism shown the Hospital by certain Philadelphia politicians. Since only the property held by the Hospital in 1816 was tax exempt, the status of subsequent Hospital real estate acquisitions was questionable. The act of 1845 expanded the exemption to all property of the Hospital.

6. Hinshaw, *Encyclopedia of American Quaker Genealogy,* II passim; Morton and Woodbury, *History of the Pennsylvania Hospital,* passim; Wood, *An Address on the Occasion of the Centennial Celebration of the Founding of the Pennsylvania Hospital* (Philadelphia, 1851), 55.

7. Morton and Woodbury, *History of the Pennsylvania Hospital,* passim; Warner, *The Private City,* 115.

8. Extracts of Wills, 64, Pennsylvania Hospital Archives; Bd. of M.M., VIII, 75, 277, 544, 759; IX, 78; Wood, *An Address on the Occasion of the Centennial Celebration of the Founding of the Pennsylvania Hospital,* 33; Morton and Woodbury, *History of the Pennsylvania Hospital,* 211; Malin, *Some Account of the Pennsylvania Hospital,* 3.

9. Extracts of Wills, Pennsylvania Hospital Archives; Morton and Woodbury, *History of the Pennsylvania Hospital,* passim; Simpson, *Lives of Eminent Philadelphians Now Deceased,* 923. An examination of Simpson, *Lives of Eminent Philadelphians Now Deceased,* Winslow, *Biographies of Successful Philadelphia Merchants* and the *D.A.B.,* finds about the same percentage of Managers listed in these volumes for the period 1801–1841, as for the period 1783–1801.

10. Bd. of M.M., VII, 277; Wood, *An Address on the Occasion of the Centennial Celebration of the Founding of the Pennsylvania Hospital,* passim; Smith, *Fiscal History of the Pennsylvania Hospital,* not paginated.

11. Wood, *An Address on the Occasion of the Centennial Celebration of the Founding of the Pennsylvania Hospital,* passim; Bd. of M.M., passim.

12. Benjamin West, *Christ Healing the Sick* (Philadelphia, 1817) 82–92; Bd. of M.M., VII, 426; Morton and Woodbury, *History of the Pennsylvania Hospital,* 305–307. West based his proposed painting on Matthew, 21, verses 14 and 15: "And the blind and the lame came to Him in the Temple; and he healed them. And when the chief priests and scribes saw the wonderful thing that He did, and the children crying in the Temple, and saying Hozanna to the son of David, they were sore displeased."

13. West, *Christ Healing the Sick,* 92–112; Bd. of M.M., VIII, 178.

14. Morton and Woodbury, *History of the Pennsylvania Hospital,* 308–312; West, *Christ Healing the Sick,* 112–128; Bd. of M.M., VIII, 240, 245, 261, 264, 265, 280–286, 291, 294. For letters from Samuel Coates to B. West see Letter Book, 1786–1828, passim, Archives of Pennsylvania Hospital. Both the British and U.S. governments cooperated by allowing the painting to be exported and imported, respectively, duty free. The most complete pamphlet on the painting was written in 1818 by John Robinson, London portrait artist. One of the mysteries concerning the West donation was that he promised, in a letter dated March 2, 1817 and reproduced in Morton and Woodbury, *History of the Pennsylvania Hospital,* 310, 311, that two other paintings were being prepared to accompany his gift of "Christ in the Temple." Nothing more has been said about the two additional paintings and there is no record that the Hospital ever received them.

15. Bd. of M.M., VIII, 285; Smith, Summary of Fiscal History of Pennsylvania

Hospital, 1800–1845, Pennsylvania Hospital Archives, not paginated; West, *Christ Healing the Sick*, 13–21.

16. Bd. of M.M., VII, 412; State of Accounts of the Pennsylvania Hospital, April 24, 1841, Archives of Pennsylvania Hospital.

17. Bd. of M.M., VII, 366; VIII, 27, 28, 84, 126, 196, 360, 361, 428, 441, 504; Morton and Woodbury, *History of Pennsylvania Hospital*, 226–232; Eaton, *New England Hospitals, 1790–1833*, 24.

18. Morton and Woodbury, *History of the Pennsylvania Hospital*, 232–234. A few births were recorded in the Hospital during the eighteenth century but the admission of pregnant women, unless they were suffering from an admittable affliction, was generally precluded prior to 1803.

19. Duffy, *A History of Public Health in New York City, 1625–1866* (New York, 1968), 253; Morton and Woodbury, *History of the Pennsylvania Hospital*, 459, 236, 237; Bd. of M.M., VII, 467, 469; VIII, 85–87. The First Troop originally intended the grant to support a foundling hospital but was persuaded by the Managers to allow all of the stock to be used to support the lying-in department.

20. Bd. of M.M., VIII, 160, 268, 269, 514, 517, 527, 535, 536; IX, 13, 28.

21. Bd. of M.M., VII, 418, 422; VIII, 97, 102, 269; Malin, *Some Account of the Pennsylvania Hospital*, 16. The out-patient department would be reopened in 1872.

22. Bd. of M.M., VII, 434, 435, 472; VIII, 21, 22, 240, 242.

23. Bd. of M.M., VIII, 286–290, 400, 419; IX, 22; Morton and Woodbury, *History of the Pennsylvania Hospital*, 82–84.

24. Bd. of M.M., VIII, 408, 421.

25. Bd. of M.M., VIII, 460–462, 465, 466; Rough Minutes, March 5, 1828, April 28, 1828; Attending Managers Minutes, November 27, 1827, February 23, 1828, May 24, 1828.

26. Malin, *Some Account of the Pennsylvania Hospital*, 19; Wood, *An Address on the Occasion of the Centennial Celebration of the Founding of the Pennsylvania Hospital*, 43; Bd. of M.M., VIII, 442.

27. Bd. of M.M., VIII, 522, 529, 530, 549; IX, 6, 34, 39–42, 44–47, 49–51, 58–60, 62, 98, 107; Morton and Woodbury, *History of the Pennsylvania Hospital*, 115–124, 165. George B. Tatum, "Architecture and Medicine in Philadelphia," *The Art of Philadelphia Medicine*, editor not given (Philadelphia, 1965), 119–121; William Stark, *Remarks on Public Hospitals for the Cure of Mental Derangement* (Edinburgh, 1807), 29. Holden's plans for the main building are not extant. Candee, Philadelphia Hospital Design, 23, 35–38. Elevations and other plans for the aborted hospital for the physically ill, were submitted by a number of noted architects and are still extant in the Pennsylvania Hospital's archives at Eighth and Pine.

28. J. Randolph, *A Memoir on the Life of Philip Syng Physick* (Philadelphia, 1839), 38; Shryock, *Medicine and Society in America: 1660–1860*, 121; Bd. of M.M., VIII, 353, 354.

29. Bd. of M.M., VII, 422; VIII, 100, 326.

30. *Ibid.*, VIII, 121, 122, 153, 210, 211, 231, 342, 377; Morton and Woodbury, *History of the Pennsylvania Hospital*, 520, 481.

31. Bd. of Managers Letter Book, 89–90; Malin, Sketch of the History of the Medical Library of the Pennsylvania Hospital, unpublished, 1830, passim; Shryock, *Medicine and Society in America: 1660–1860*, 153; Bd. of M.M., VII and VIII, passim; Morton and Woodbury, *History of the Pennsylvania Hospital*, 349; Bell, "The Old Library of the Pennsylvania Hospital," *Bulletin of the Medical Library Association* (October, 1972), 548–549.

32. Bd. of M.M., VII, 476; VIII, 46–49.

33. *Ibid.*, VIII, 30, 100, 121, 122, 321, 326, 343, 344, 379, 392, 418, 419, 486; Morton and Woodbury, *History of the Pennsylvania Hospital*, 535, 536.

34. Bd. of M.M., VII, 506; VIII, 345, 460, 116, 191, 200–201, 203, 205, 224, 429.

35. *Ibid.*, VIII, 203, 205, 224, 429, 436.

36. *Ibid.*, VIII, 437, 346, 405, 424, 483, 485, 509.

37. *Ibid.*, VIII, 509, 448, 449, 513; IX, 27, 32, 36, 66; VIII,566.

38. Bd. of M.M., VIII, 333, 398, 516; IX, 67, 130; Morton and Woodbury, *History of the Pennsylvania Hospital*, 540–544. A copy of Malin's history of the library is in the Hospital archives at Eighth and Pine.

39. Bd. of M.M., VIII, 498; IX, 130; Summary of Attending Managers Monthly Reports, 1814–1822, 1822–1825, passim; Malin, *Some Account of the Pennsylvania Hospital*, 21.

40. Annual Reports, Archives of Pennsylvania Hospital, passim.

41. Bd. of M.M., VII, 511; VIII, 17, 114, 275, 562. On his visit to the Philadelphia Almshouse (Bettering House) in 1788, J. P. Brissot de Warville noted that blacks and whites were lodged in the same apartments and wards. Since the Almshouse was run by Quakers at this time, it can be assumed that integration of blacks and whites was also carried on at Eighth and Pine during the eighteenth century. By 1827, however, the segregation of blacks was the official policy at Eighth and Pine. Bd. of M.M., VIII, 449, 483; Warville, *New Travels in the U.S. of North America*, ed., Echeverria, 176; Morton and Woodbury, *History of the Pennsylvania Hospital*, 212; William G. Malin, *Some Account of the Pennsylvania Hospital* (Philadelphia, 1831), 8, 12.

42. James Mease, *Picture of Philadelphia from 1811 to 1831* (Philadelphia, 1831), 229–235; Bd. of M.M., VIII, 150, and passim; David Sears to Dr. John C. Warren, January 6, 1821, Warren Papers, Vol. IX, Massachusetts Historical Society; Malin, *Some Account of the Pennsylvania Hospital*, 20–21.

43. Morton and Woodbury, *History of the Pennsylvania Hospital*, 453–455; Bd. of M.M., VIII, 253.

44. Thomas G. Morton, *Surgery in the Pennsylvania Hospital* (Philadelphia, 1880), 137–138; David Sears to Dr. John C. Warren, January 6, 1821, Warren Papers, Vol. IX, Massachusetts Historical Society. For a detailed look at some of the surgical techniques and their results see Patients Hospital Cases, I, 1803–1828, Historical Library, Pennsylvania Hospital.

45. J. Howe Adams, *History of the Life of D. Hayes Agnew* (Philadelphia, 1892), 47. For more information on the Hospital's operating room during this period see Alfred R. Henderson, "A Note on the Circular Room of the Pennsylvania Hospital," *Journal of the Medicine and Allied Service*, Vol. XIX, 1964, 156–160.

46. Bd. of M.M., VII, passim; VIII, 163–167, 193, 370, passim; IX, 2; Morton and Woodbury, *History of the Pennsylvania Hospital*, 121–122, 178, 179.

47. Morton and Woodbury, *History of the Pennsylvania Hospital*, 122; John Duffy, *A History of Public Health in New York City*, 243, 245.

48. Leonard K. Eaton, *New England Hospitals, 1790–1833*, 212, 213.

Selective Bibliography

Primary Sources

Unprinted Documents, Diaries and Letters:

Archives of Pennsylvania Hospital, Eighth and Pine Streets, Philadelphia, Pennsylvania. Of particular value were:

1. Board of Managers Minutes, 1751–1841.
2. Board of Managers Minutes (Rough), 1781–1841.
3. Attending Managers Accounts, 1752–1841.
4. Treasurer's Cash Books and Ledgers, 1752–1841.
5. Stewards' and Matrons' cash books, 1754–1756, 1758–1760, 1761–1841.

Most of the early papers of the Pennsylvania Hospital have been microfilmed and can be seen at the American Philosophical Society Library in Philadelphia.

COATES, SAMUEL. Samuel Coates Letter Book, Coates-Reynell Papers. Philadelphia: Historical Society of Pennsylvania.

MEMORANDUM BOOK OF SAMUEL COATES. Historical Library, Pennsylvania Hospital.

PEMBERTON COPY BOOK, 1740–1780, PEMBERTON PAPERS. Philadelphia: Historical Society of Pennsylvania.

PEMBERTON PAPERS, ETTING COLLECTION. Philadelphia: Historical Society of Pennsylvania.

PENN MANUSCRIPTS, OFFICIAL CORRESPONDENCE. Philadelphia: Historical Society of Pennsylvania.

PENN, THOMAS. Thomas Penn's Letter Book. Philadelphia: Historical Society of Pennsylvania.

PETERS, RICHARD. Manuscript Letters from Thomas Penn to Richard Peters and Others, 1752–1772, Peters' Papers. Philadelphia: Historical Society of Pennsylvania.

RUSH, BENJAMIN. Correspondence of Doctor Benjamin Rush. Library Company Collection. Philadelphia: Historical Society of Pennsylvania.

SMITH, JOHN. John Smith's Diaries. Library Company Collection. Philadelphia: Historical Society of Pennsylvania.

Printed Documents, Diaries, Letters, Magazines, Newspapers, Reports and Sermons.

An Account of the Rise, Progress and Present State of the Pennsylvania Hospital. Philadelphia: Robert Carr, 1801.

An Account of the Public Hospital for the Diseased Poor in the County of York. York, England: 1743.

An Account of the Rise and Establishment of the Infirmary, or the Hospital for the Sick-poor, Erected at Edinburgh, 1730.

BRIDENBAUGH, CARL. "Dr. Thomas Bond's Essay on the Utility of Clinical Lectures," *Journal of the History of Medicine and Allied Sciences,* II (1949), 10–19.

CLARK, ALURED. *A Collection of Papers Relating to the County Hospital for Sick and Lame at Winchester.* London: J. J. Pemberton, 1737. *A Sermon Preached in the Cathedral Church at Winchester.* London: J. J. Pemberton, 1937. *A Proposal for Erecting a Public Hospital,* is attached to the back of Clark's other two works and found in the historical library of Wellcome Institute, London.

Continuation Account of the Pennsylvania Hospital from First of May 1754 to the Fifth of May, 1761. Philadelphia: B. Franklin and D. Hall, 1761.

DODDRIDGE, P. *Compassion to the Sick Recommended and Urged.* London: 1743.

FRANKLIN, BENJAMIN. *The Autobiography and Other Writings.* L. Jesse Lemisch, ed. New York: New American Library of World Literature, Inc., 1961.

————. *Some Account of the Pennsylvania Hospital,* I. Bernard Cohen, ed. Baltimore: Johns Hopkins Press, 1954.

GREY, RICHARD. *A Sermon for the Sick and Lame at Northampton County Infirmary.* Northampton: 1744.

HOWARD, JOHN. *An Account of the Principal Lazarettos in Europe.* London: William Eyres, 1789.

————. *The State of the Prisons in England and Wales with Preliminary Observations and an Account of Some Foreign Prisons and Hospitals.* London: William Eyres, 1780.

HOLME, THOMAS. *A Sermon.* Northampton, England: 1745.

HONYMAN, ROBERT. *Colonial Panorama, 1775.* Philip Padelford, ed. San Marino, California: Huntington Library, 1939.

ISAAC, LORD BISHOP OF ST. ATAPH. *The Duties and Advantages of Encouraging Public Infirmaries: A Sermon.* London: 1743.

JOHN, LORD BISHOP OF PETERBOROUGH. *A Sermon.* Northampton, England: 1748.

Letter from a Gentleman in Town to His Friend in the Country Relating to the Royal Infirmary in Edinburgh. Edinburgh: 1749.

LAYNG, HENRY. *A Sermon.* Northampton, England: 1746.

NIXON, JOHN. *A Sermon.* Northampton: 1749.

RUSH, BENJAMIN. *The Autobiography of Benjamin Rush.* George W. Corner, ed. Westport, Connecticut: Greenwood Press, 1948.

————. *The Letters of Benjamin Rush,* I, II. L. H. Butterfield, ed. Princeton: American Philosophical Society and Princeton University Press, 1951.

Secondary Sources

Unpublished:

CANDEE, RICHARD. Philadelphia Hospital Design, 1754–1844. An unpublished course paper. Philadelphia: University of Pennsylvania. A copy is available at the office of Miss Joyce Cooper of the Pennsylvania Hospital.

HYSLOP, NEWTON E., JR. London Hospitals in the Eighteenth Century. Senior honors thesis. Cambridge, Massachusetts: Harvard, 1957.

MALIN, WILLIAM G. Sketch of the History of the Medical Library of the Pennsylvania Hospital. Philadelphia: Historical Society of Pennsylvania.

SMITH, GEORGE ROBERTS. Summary of Fiscal History of [Pennsylvania] Hospital. Philadelphia: Pennsylvania Hospital Archives, Pennsylvania Hospital, Eighth and Pine, 1844.

Published Works:

ABEL-SMITH, BRIAN. *The Hospital Movement of England and Wales, 1800–1948.* Cambridge, Massachusetts: Harvard University Press, 1964.

BELL, WHITFIELD, JR. "James Hutchinson (1752–1793), A Physician in Politics," *Medicine, Science and Culture,* 265–283.

_____. *John Morgan, Continental Doctor.* Philadelphia: University of Pennsylvania Press, 1965.

_____. "The Old Library of the Pennsylvania Hospital," *Bulletin of the Medical Library Association,* October 1972, 543–550.

_____. "Thomas Parke's Student Life in England and Scotland, 1771–1773," *Pennsylvania Magazine of History and Biography,* LXXV (1951), 237–258.

_____. "Some Aspects of the Social History of Pennsylvania, 1760–1790," *Pennsylvania Magazine of History and Biography,* LXII (1938), 281–308.

BIDDLE, HENRY. "Colonial Mayors of Philadelphia; Samuel Rhoads," *Pennsylvania Magazine of History and Biography,* XIX (1895), 64–71.

BINGER, CARL. *Revolutionary Doctor: Benjamin Rush, 1746–1813.* New York: W. W. Norton and Co., Inc., 1966.

BRIDENBAUGH, CARL and JESSICA. *Rebels and Gentlemen: Philadelphia in the Age of Franklin.* New York: Oxford University Press, 1962.

CLARK-KENNEDY, A. E. *The London, A Study in the Voluntary Hospital System,* I. London: Pitman Medical Publishing Co., 1962.

CORNER, GEORGE W. *Two Centuries of Medicine, A History of the School of Medicine, University of Pennsylvania.* Philadelphia: Lippincott, 1965.

CROSKEY, JOHN WELSH. *History of Blockley.* Philadelphia: F. A. Davis Co., 1929.

DAINTON, COURTNEY. *The Story of the England's Hospitals.* Springfield, Illinois: Charles C. Thomas, 1961.

DEUTSCH, ALBERT. *The Mentally Ill in America,* 2nd ed. New York: Columbia University Press, 1960.

DOWNIE, ROBERT W. "Pennsylvania Hospital Admissions, 1751–1850: A Survey," *Transactions and Studies of the College of Physicians of Philadelphia,* XXXII (1964-65), 21–35.

EATON, LEONARD K. *New England Hospitals, 1790–1833.* Ann Arbor: University of Michigan Press, 1957.

_____. "Medicine in Philadelphia and Boston, 1805–1830, *Pennsylvania Magazine of History and Biography,* LXXV.

FOX, R. HINGSTON. *Dr. John Fothergill and His Friends.* London: Macmillan and Co., 1919.

GROB, GERALD N. *The State and the Mentally Ill, A History of Worcester State Hospital in Massachusetts, 1830–1920.* Chapel Hill: University of North Carolina Press, 1966.

_____. *Mental Institutions in America, Social Policy to 1875.* New York: Free Press, 1973.

HANNA, WILLIAM S. *Benjamin Franklin and Pennsylvania Politics.* Stanford, California: Stanford University Press, 1964.

HEFFNER, WILLIAM CLINTON. *History of Poor Relief Legislation in Pennsylvania, 1682–1913.* Cleona, Pennsylvania: Holzapfel Publishing Co., 1912.

JAMES, SYDNEY A. *A People Among Peoples: Quaker Benevolence in Eighteenth Century Philadelphia.* Cambridge, Massachusetts: Harvard University Press, 1963.

JERNEGAN, MARCUS W. *Laboring and Dependent Classes in Colonial America.* Chicago: University of Chicago, 1931.

Jones, Rufus M. *The Quakers in the American Colonies.* New York: W. W. Norton and Company, 1966.

Kelly, Howard A.; Burrage, Walter L. *Dictionary of American Medical Biography.* New York: D. Appleton and Co., 1928.

Krumbhaar, Edward. "The Pennsylvania Hospital," *Historic Philadelphia.* Luther Eisenhart, ed. Philadelphia: American Philosophical Society, 1953.

Lawrence, Charles. *History of the Philadelphia Almshouses and Hospitals.* Philadelphia: C. Lawrence, 1905.

Larrabee, Eric. *The Benevolent and Necessary Institution, The New York Hospital, 1771–1791.* New York: Doubleday & Co., 1971.

Malin, William G. *Some Account of the Pennsylvania Hospital, Its Origin, Objects and Present State.* Philadelphia: Thomas Kiet, 1831.

McMenemey, W. H. "The Hospital Movement of the Eighteenth Century and Its Development," *The Evolution of Hospitals in Britain.* F. N. L. Poynter, ed. London: Pittman Medical Publishing Co., 1964.

Morton, Thomas G., and Woodbury, Frank. *History of the Pennsylvania Hospital, 1751–1895.* Philadelphia: Times Printing Press, 1897.

Packard, Francis R. "Medical Case Histories in a Colonial Hospital," *Bulletin of the History of Medicine,* XII (1940), 145–168.

————. *Some Account of the Pennsylvania Hospital from 1751 to 1938.* Philadelphia: Engle Press, 1938.

Rothman, David J. *The Discovery of the Asylum.* Boston: Little, Brown and Co., 1971.

Russell, William L. *The New York Hospital, A History of Psychiatric Service 1771–1936.* New York: Columbia University Press, 1945.

Shryock, Richard. *The Development of Modern Medicine.* Philadelphia: University of Pennsylvania Press, 1936.

————. *The History of Nursing.* Philadelphia: W. B. Saunders Co., 1959.

————. *Medical Licensing in America, 1650–1965.* Baltimore: Johns Hopkins Press, 1967.

————. *Medicine and Society in America, 1660–1860.* Ithaca, New York: Cornell University Press, 1962.

Smith, G. Munro. *History of the Bristol Royal Infirmary.* Bristol: J. W. Arrowsmith, Ltd., 1917.

Tatum, George B. "Architecture and Medicine in Philadelphia," *The Art of Philadelphia Medicine.* Philadelphia Museum of Art, 1965.

Thacher, James. *American Medical Biography.* Boston: Richardson and Lord, 1828.

Thayer, Theodore. *Israel Pemberton: King of the Quakers.* Philadelphia: Historical Society of Pennsylvania, 1943.

Thomson, Elizabeth. "Thomas Bond, 1713–1784: First Professor of Clinical Medicine in the American Colonies," *Journal of Medical Education,* XXXIII, 9 (September, 1959), 614–624.

Turner, A. Logan. *Story of a Great Hospital, The Royal Infirmary of Edinburgh, 1729–1929.* London: Oliver and Boyd, 1937.

Warner, Sam Bass. *The Private City: Philadelphia in Three Periods of Its Growth.* Philadelphia: University of Pennsylvania Press, 1970.

West, Benjamin. *Christ Healing the Sick.* Philadelphia: James Webster, 1817.

Wood, George B. *An Address on the Occasion of the Centennial Celebration of the Founding of the Pennsylvania Hospital.* Philadelphia: T. K. and P. G. Colins, 1851.

Index